Hepatology Research and Clinical Developments

AF696694

Acute Cholecystitis

Diagnosis, Management and Complications

HEPATOLOGY RESEARCH AND CLINICAL DEVELOPMENTS

Additional books in this series can be found on Nova's website under the Series tab.

Additional e-books in this series can be found on Nova's website under the e-book tab.

HEPATOLOGY RESEARCH AND CLINICAL DEVELOPMENTS

ACUTE CHOLECYSTITIS

DIAGNOSIS, MANAGEMENT AND COMPLICATIONS

LISA POWELL
EDITOR

New York

Library of Congress Cataloging-in-Publication Data

Library of Congress Control Number: 2016945954
ISBN: 978-1-63485-744-4

Published by Nova Science Publishers, Inc. † New York

CONTENTS

PREFACE

Acute cholecystitis is a pathological entity of inflammatory origin, with a high prevalence worldwide. The term cholecystitis defines an inflammation of the gallbladder. Although most people with gallstones do not have symptoms and will not go on to develop cholecystitis, cholecystitis occurs most commonly due to blockage of the cystic duct with gallstones (cholelithiasis). In this book, Chapter One provides a contemporary review of acute cholecystitis (AC). Chapter Two examines the diagnosis and treatment options for AC. Chapter Three focuses on the diagnostic work-up of patients with AC. Chapter Four discusses early and delayed cholecystectomy as a treatment for AC. Chapter Five examines the current literature as it pertains to the management of patients who present with Grade II (moderate) acute cholecystitis, specifically looking at the timing of operation and the appropriateness of drainage procedures. Chapter Six reviews cholecystitis in systemic lupus erythematosus.

Chapter 1 - Acute cholecystitis predominantly occurs as a complication of gallstone disease (90 per cent of all cases); on the other hand, Acalculous Cholecystitis (10 per cent of all cases) develops almost in critically ill patients (risk factors: surgery, trauma, burn, and parenteral nutrition).

Diagnosis: Acute cholecystitis should be suspected in a patient presenting with right upper quadrant or epigastric pain, positive Murphy's sign, fever and leukocytosis. Confirmation of diagnosis requires demonstration of gallbladder wall thickening or edema or a sonographic Murphy's sign; abdominal ultrasound should be performed to confirm the diagnosis.

Management: Patients with acute cholecystitis should be admitted to the hospital for supportive care, which includes intravenous fluid therapy, correction of electrolyte disorders, and control of pain. Antibiotics may also be indicated. The selection and timing of definitive therapy depends upon the severity of symptoms and the patient's overall risk for cholecystectomy. If gangrene or perforation are suspected, or if the patient develops progressive symptoms and signs such as fever, hemodynamic instability, or intractable pain while on supportive therapy, emergency cholecystectomy or gallbladder drainage may be needed. Low-risk patients without emergent indications for operation generally undergo laparoscopic cholecystectomy preferably during the same admission. High-risk patients without emergent indications for surgeryare treated with a gallbladder drainage procedure if symptoms do not improve with supportive care. For patients whose medical status can be optimized to allow surgery, cholecystectomy can be considered.

Complications: Left untreated, symptoms of cholecystitis may appear within 7 to 10 days. The most common complication is the development of *gallbladder gangrene* (up to 20 percent of cases) with subsequent perforation (2 percent of cases). *Perforation* is often localized, resulting in a pericholecystic abscess; otherwise, perforation could be free into the peritoneum, leading to generalized peritonitis. Less common complications are *cholecystoenteric fistula, gallstone ileus* (mechanical bowel obstruction caused by the passage of a gallstone through a cholecystoenteric fistula)and *Emphysematous cholecystitis*(secondary infection of the gallbladder wall with gas-forming organisms, such as Escherichia Coli, *Clostridium welchii, staphylococci, streptococci, Pseudomonas,* and *Klebsiella.*

Chapter 2 - Acute cholecystitis is a common emergency presentation of gallstone disease. The improvements in diagnosis and treatment can lead to reduce rates of morbidity, mortality and costs.

Clinical findings are usually diagnostic of acute cholecystitis. However, imaging studies play an important role in the confirmation of the diagnosis and detection of associated complications.

On physical examination patients typically present severe right upper quadrant pain with positive Murphy sign associated with nausea, vomits and fever. Leukocytosis with neutrophilia is the most common laboratory finding, while elevated liver enzymes are related with worse outcome.

Imaging studies allow clinicians to establish diagnosis in suspected individuals and to detect complications. Right upper quadrant ultrasound is the imaging modality of choice due to its sensitivity (82%), specificity (81%), availability, low cost and lack of radiation exposure. Computed Tomography (CT) is currently recommended when other intraabdominal pathologies are suspected and Magnetic Resonance Imaging (MRI) is useful for pregnant patients and to identify choledocholithiasis.

Once the diagnosis of acute cholecystitis is achieved, the authors must take decisions in order to provide patients the best management available. Despite of overtime controverses about the optimal treatment, early laparoscopic cholecystectomy is currently accepted as the best option. Surgery should be performed as soon as possible after diagnosis, because it reduces total hospital stay and does not increase complication or conversion rates. Percutaneous cholecystostomy is indicated in the advanced form of inflammation or in patients with severe comorbidities increasing surgical risk.

Chapter 3 - *Introduction:* The diagnosis of acute cholecystitis (AC) can be challenging, may result in misdiagnosis, patient's hospital discharge without operation, delay in cholecystectomy and increased mortality. To improve accuracy in the diagnosis of AC, the 2007 and 2013 Tokyo guidelines (TG07/TG13) added elevated concentration of C-reactive protein (CRP) as one of the analytic criteria. However, CRP is not widely used for diagnosing AC and its grade of severity. To determine the utility of CRP in the diagnosis of AC, the discriminative power of CRP was compared with that of white cell count (WCC) in patients with AC of different histological grades of severity. The authors found that CRP had a better discriminative power than WCC in predicting the histological severity of AC including acute on chronic, acute edematous, necrotizing, suppurative and gangrenous cholecystitis. The authors suggest that leucopenia (WCC $< 4000/mm^3$) and combinations of systemic signs of inflammation should be added to modify the Tokyo diagnostic criteria for AC. Patients with acute on chronic and acute edematous cholecystitis had low rates of CTO and were therefore included in the mild category of AC. Patients with acute necrotizing, suppurative, gangrenous cholecystitis, pericholecystic abscess and AC with gallbladder perforation were allocated to the moderate - severe category of AC and these were associated with a twofold increased risk of CTO.

Conclusion: Tokyo diagnostic criteria for AC should be modified to include combinations of more than one systemic sign of inflammation as indicators of severity, and, leucopenia should be added as an analytic criterion.

Chapter 4 - Acute cholecystitis is a pathological entity of inflammatory origin, with a high prevalence worldwide. Therefore, an appropriate diagnostic and therapeutic approach has important medical and socio-economic impact. There are two different alternatives for the surgical management of acute cholecystitis: early cholecystectomy during the index admission, within 72 hours from the onset of symptoms if possible, or delayed cholecystectomy during a later scheduled admission 4-6 weeks after a successful conservative treatment. Early cholecystectomy reduces days of hospital stay, hospital readmissions and seems to lead to a reduction in direct hospital costs. Only 50% of patients from delayed cholecystectomy will get their elective operation after the index episode, leaving half of the cases at risk of complications and mortality. Laparoscopic approach seems to be as safe as open surgery. Subtotal cholecystectomy may have the advantage of avoiding bile duct injury, and could decrease conversions rate in laparoscopic procedures.

Chapter 5 - Acute cholecystitis is a common sequelae of cholelithiasis that is encountered in surgical practices worldwide. It varies in severity, causing minimal discomfort in otherwise healthy individuals to being potentially fatal in the critically ill or those with significant comorbidities. In the US alone, it is estimated 500,000 cholecystectomies are performed per year, with an unknown percentage being done for acute cholecystitis. In Japan, the number of cases of acute cholecystitis in a nearly 15 year period had increased from 3.9 million to over 10 million.

Despite being a common and increasingly surgical problem, prior to ten years ago there were no accepted standards for the diagnostic criteria, severity assessment, or management of acute cholecystitis. In 2006, an International Consensus Meeting took place in Tokyo, Japan, where international experts in the field combined personal expertise with evidence based data to create the Tokyo Guidelines, with a revision following in 2013. These guidelines not only assist in making a diagnosis, but provide an algorithm for the management of acute cholecystitis based on severity, or a determined grade. This grade is formulated based upon presenting symptoms, clinical picture, laboratory values, and imaging results. Grade I (mild) acute cholecystitis describes patients with limited or early gallbladder disease and no organ dysfunction. Grade II (moderate) acute cholecystitis describes patients with extensive gallbladder disease and no organ dysfunction. Finally, Grade III (severe) acute cholecystitis describes patients with extensive gallbladder disease and organ dysfunction.

Although cholecystectomy has been the standard of care for the management of acute cholecystitis, the timing, approach, and necessity of a drainage procedure have all have been at the forefront of academic contention. With the introduction and adoption of the Tokyo Guidelines, one would expect these "controversies" to come to rest. While the majority of cases fall into Grade I or III (75%), it is the remaining 25% that prompt a detailed examination of the literature regarding optimal management. For grades I and III acute cholecystitis, management is well established, with laparoscopic cholecystectomy for grade I and antibiotics with early drainage for grade III. On the contrary, Grade II or moderate acute cholecystitis, poses the greatest management dilemma, as its clinical presentation allows for the most variability. In this chapter the authors examine the current literature as it pertains to the management of patients who present with Grade II (moderate) acute cholecystitis, specifically looking at the timing of operation and the appropriateness of drainage procedures.

Chapter 6 - Gastrointestinal (GI) manifestations of systemic lupus erythematosus (SLE) are common. Any part of the GI tract can be involved but cholecystitis is rare in SLE patients. Only a few cases are reported. Cholecystitis can be an initial manifestation of SLE or can occur in the disease course, in association with other severe involvements. Clinical presentation is non-specific. Patients have abdominal pain, vomiting and fever. Examination can reveal right upper quadrant tenderness. Symptoms can be attenuated by the use of corticosteroid when patients are already treated for SLE. Laboratory data can show increased level of liver enzymes. Ultrasonography may show gallbladder thickness wall with or without pericholecystic edema and in most of cases, there are no signs of lithiasis. Abdominal computed tomography confirms the diagnosis showing gallbladder wall thickness and edema.

When cholecystectomy is performed, histological examination confirms the inflammation and in most cases shows vasculitis which can be associated with fibrinoid necrosis. Otherwise, thromboembolic events with or without antiphospholipid antibodies can be responsible for acute cholecystitis.

In the absence of controlled trials, treatment of acalculous cholecystitis is based on clinical experiences. High dose steroid may be the first line therapy but other immunosuppressant agents (cyclophosphamide, azathiorpine) can be considered. Anticoagulants are used when thrombosis is identified as a cause. Cholecystectomy is often performed in patients when cholecystitis inaugurates the disease and SLE is not yet diagnosed. In other cases, patients may undergo surgery when medical treatment is ineffective.

In: Acute Cholecystitis
Editor: Lisa Powell

ISBN: 978-1-63485-744-4

Chapter 1

ACUTE CHOLECYSTITIS: A CONTEMPORARY REVIEW

Edgardo Picardi, Valeria Valli, Gioia Pozza and Cosimo Sperti*
Department of Surgery, Oncology and Gastroenterology, University of Padua, Padua, Italy

ABSTRACT

Acute cholecystitis predominantly occurs as a complication of gallstone disease (90 per cent of all cases); on the other hand, Acalculous Cholecystitis (10 per cent of all cases) develops almost in critically ill patients (risk factors: surgery, trauma, burn, and parenteral nutrition).

Diagnosis: Acute cholecystitis should be suspected in a patient presenting with right upper quadrant or epigastric pain, positive Murphy's sign, fever and leukocytosis. Confirmation of diagnosis requires demonstration of gallbladder wall thickening or edema or a sonographic Murphy's sign; abdominal ultrasound should be performed to confirm the diagnosis.

Management: Patients with acute cholecystitis should be admitted to the hospital for supportive care, which includes intravenous fluid therapy, correction of electrolyte disorders, and control of pain. Antibiotics may also be indicated. The selection and timing of definitive therapy depends upon the severity of symptoms and the patient's overall risk for

* Corresponding author: Email: cosimo.sperti@unipd.it.

cholecystectomy. If gangrene or perforation are suspected, or if the patient develops progressive symptoms and signs such as fever, hemodynamic instability, or intractable pain while on supportive therapy, emergency cholecystectomy or gallbladder drainage may be needed. Low-risk patients without emergent indications for operation generally undergo laparoscopic cholecystectomy preferably during the same admission. High-risk patients without emergent indications for surgeryare treated with a gallbladder drainage procedure if symptoms do not improve with supportive care. For patients whose medical status can be optimized to allow surgery, cholecystectomy can be considered.

Complications: Left untreated, symptoms of cholecystitis may appear within 7 to 10 days. The most common complication is the development of *gallbladder gangrene* (up to 20 percent of cases) with subsequent perforation (2 percent of cases). *Perforation* is often localized, resulting in a pericholecystic abscess; otherwise, perforation could be free into the peritoneum, leading to generalized peritonitis. Less common complications are *cholecystoenteric fistula, gallstone ileus* (mechanical bowel obstruction caused by the passage of a gallstone through a cholecystoenteric fistula) and *Emphysematous cholecystitis*(secondary infection of the gallbladder wall with gas-forming organisms, such as Escherichia Coli, *Clostridium welchii, staphylococci, streptococci, Pseudomonas,* and *Klebsiella.*

Keywords:acute cholecystitis, gallbladder, gallstones, cholecystectomy, cholecystostomy

Acute Calculous Cholecystitis

Acute cholecystitis is defined as inflammation of gallbladder and results from obstruction of the cystic duct or Hartmann's pouch with gallstones (90-95% of cases) leading to painful gallbladder distension; Acalculous Cholecystitis amounts for the remnant 10% of all acute cholecystitis (Hafif 1991, Lillemoe 2000, Friedman 1993, Shapiro 1994). The duration of cystic duct obstruction is the primary pathophysiology phenomenon that contributes to the evolution of the inflammatory process. As the gallbladder becomes distended, blood flow and lymphatic drainage are compromised, leading to first edema and subserosal hemorrhage, then polymorphonuclear (PMN) leukocytes appear. Secondary bacterial contamination is reported in 15 to 30% of patients undergoing cholecystectomy for acute uncomplicated cholecystitis. In the cases without resolution of the obstruction, the gallbladder will progress to mucosal ischemia and necrosis (5-10% of cases), secondary bacterial infection, with subsequent complications: empyema, gangrene, contained or free perforation of the gallbladder with abscess formation.

The toxic action on the gallbladder wall caused by the imprisoned bile salts contributes to the pathophysiology of acute cholecystitis: lipids may penetrate the Rokitansky-Aschoff sinuses causing an irritant reaction, and the inflammatory process is probably also mediated by the mucosal toxin lysolecithin, a product of lecithin, such as platelet-activating factor. Increase in prostaglandin synthesis amplifies the inflammatory response (Roslyn 1980, Kaminski 1989). Bacteria infection result to have a minor role in the early stages of acute cholecystitis, even though most complications of the disease involve suppuration. In fact, bacterial deconjugation of bile salts may produce toxic bile acids which can injure the mucosa. Bacteria that infect the bile include gram-negative bacilli (Escherichia coli, Klebsiellaspp, Enterobacterspp), anaerobes (Bacteroides, Clostridia spp, Fusobacteriumspp) and gram-positive cocci (enterococci). Overgrowth of gas-producing bacteria within the gallbladder can lead to emphysematous cholecystitis (Johannsen 2005).

DIAGNOSIS

According to a review referring to Tokyo Guidelines diagnostic criteria of acute cholecystitis, a definite diagnosis can be made when a local sign or symptom and a systemic sign are present, and test imaging provides confirmation (Steven 2008).

Clinical Presentation

The symptoms of acute cholecystitis are similar to, but more severe than uncomplicated biliary colic. The first symptom is abdominal pain but, in contrast to biliary colic, it does not subside, it is unremitting and may persist for several days. Pain often occurs late at night or in the early morning, usually in the right upper abdomen or epigastrium and it is sometimes associated with referred pain in the region of the right scapula; the proportion of patients with right hypochondrial pain and epigastric pain combined is 72-93%. The patient is often febrile (the temperature usually ranges from 38 to 38.5°C), complains of anorexia, nausea, and vomiting (about half of patients), but the vomiting is rarely severe. Patients are more reluctant to move as the inflammatory process affects the parietal peritoneum. On physical examination, right upper quadrant tenderness is common and may be severe with localized guarding or rebound. In about a third of patients the gallbladder is palpable (often in a position lateral to its normal one); however, guarding may prevent this. Singer et al. found that a positive Murphy's sign was highly sensitive (97%) and predictive (positive predictive value 93%) of acute cholecystitis (Singer 1996): if instructed to breathe deeply during palpation in the right subcostal region, the patient experiences accentuated tenderness and sudden inspiratory arrest. This is most informative when the acute inflammation has subsided and direct tenderness is absent (Trowbridge 2003). Presentation in elderly patients may be atypical. Hafif et al. reported that among 131 patients over 70 years with acute cholecystitis, right upper quadrant pain was absent in 27% and fever was absent in 45% (Hafif 1991). Mild jaundice may be present. Severe jaundice, however, in the setting of a picture of acute cholecystitis is rare: it can be a manifestation of cholangitis, with obstruction of the common bile duct, or Mirizzi syndrome, in which inflammation or a stone in the gallbladder neck leads to inflammation of the adjacent biliary system, with obstruction of the common hepatic duct.

Laboratory Data

There are no specific blood tests for making a diagnosis of acute cholecystitis: however, the white blood cell count and the measurement of C-reactive protein (typically more than 3 mg/dl) are very useful in confirming an inflammatory process. A mild to moderate leukocytosis (typically 12,000 to 15,000 cells/mm3) is usually present. However, some patients may have a normal white blood cell count. At the same time, an high white blood cell count (more than 20,000 cells/mm3) is suggestive of a complicated form of cholecystitis such as gangrenous cholecystitis, perforation or associated cholangitis. A mild elevation of the serum bilirubin (< 4 mg/ml) is common, presumably owing to secondary inflammation of the common duct by the contiguous gallbladder. Also liver function tests, including alkaline phosphatase, gamma-glutamyltransferase (AST), alanine aminotransferase (ALT), and serum amylase can be altered (hyperamylasemia is a useful parameter to identify complications such as choledocholithiasis causing biliary pancreatitis). To assess the severity of the illness useful laboratory data are platelet count, blood urea nitrogen, creatinine, and prothrombin time (PT)

(Hirota 2007). In the febrile patient blood cultures may be positive. When ultrasonography shows findings that suggest acute cholecystitis and a C-reactive protein level exceeding 3 mg/dl, a diagnosis of acute cholecystitis can be made with 97% sensitivity, 76% specificity, and 95% positive predictive value (Juvonen 1992).

Imaging Studies

Ultrasonography (US) is the most helpful study in diagnosing acute cholecystitis. It is the test that should be performed first of all for every case of suspected acute cholecystitis (Shea 1984, Ralls 1985, Cooperberg 1980, Kalimi 2001, Chatziioannou 2000, Kiewiet 2012). On a meta-analysis of five studies involving a total of 532 cases, Shea et al. (1994) reportedthatultrasonography for acute cholecystitis showed asensitivity of 88% (95% CI 0,74-1.00) and specificity of 80% (95% CI 0.62-0.98). A diagnosis of acute calculouscholecystitis can be made radiologically when the following findings are present at the same time: thickening of the gallbladder wall (5 mm or greater if the patient does not have chronic liver disease and/or ascites or right heart failure), pericholecystic fluid, enlarged gallbladder (long axis diameter >8cm, short axis diameter >4cm) (Figure 1) or direct tenderness when the probe is pushed against the gallbladder (ultrasonographic Murphy's sign). This last finding is often absent, however, when the gallbladder is gangrenous. Other ultrasonographic findings may include gallbladder enlargement, gallbladder stones (Figure 2), debris echo (Figure 3) and gas imaging (Ralls 1985, Martinez 1986, Ralls 1982, Bree 1995).

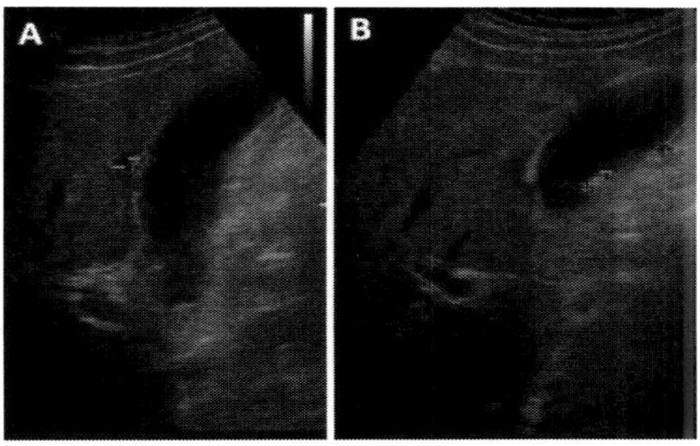

Figure 1.Ultrasonography of the abdomen showing an enlargement of the gallbladder, thickening of the wall, pericholecystic fluid (A) and gallstone (B) in a patient withacute calculouscholecystitis.

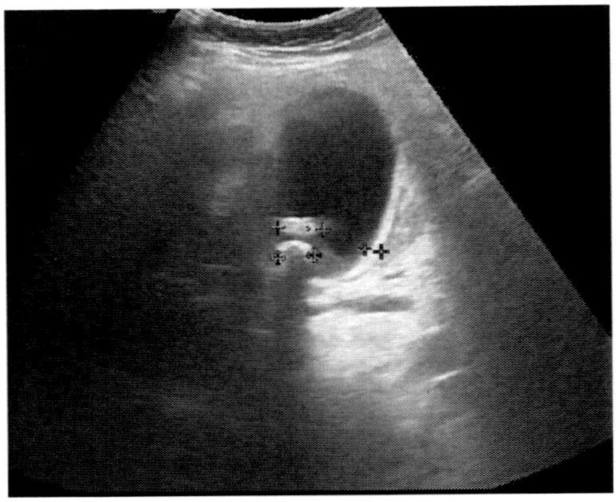

Figure 2.Ultrasonography of the abdomen showing an enlarged gallbladder with echogenic gallstone and thickened wall.

CT Scans is frequently obtained in patients with right upper quadrant pain and may also demonstrate evidence of acute cholecystitis. CT findings of acute cholecystitis were reported as: gallbladder distension (41%), gallbladder wall thickening (59%), pericholecystic fat density (52%), pericholecystic fluid collection (31%), subserosal edema (31%), and high-attenuation gallbladder bile (24%). It is worth to notice that CT is less sensitive than US (Fidler 1996).

If additional diagnostic information is desirable (i.e., if US is equivocal or negative), a radionuclide scanning (*HIDA scan*) may help. Lack of filling of the gallbladder after 4 hours indicates an obstructed cystic duct and, in the clinical setting of acute cholecystitis, is highly sensitive (sensitivity 97%) and specific (specificity 87%) (Ralls 1982).

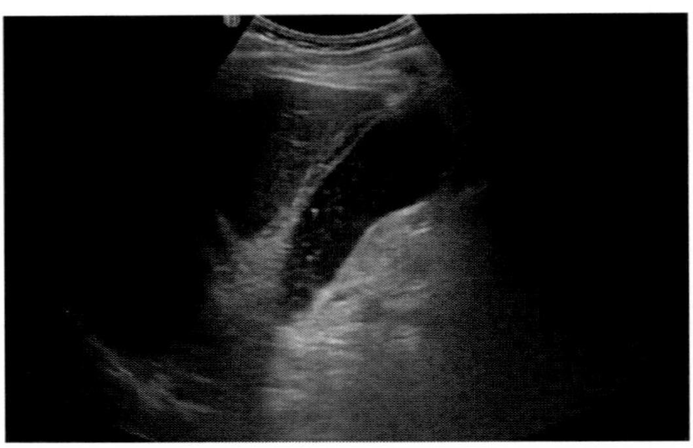

Figure 3.Ultrasonography of the gallbladder showing debris echo, thickening of thewall and pericholecystic fluid.

Patients with acute cholecystitis may present with a spectrum of disease stages ranging from a mild, self-limited illness to a fulminant, potentially life-threatening illness.

The severity assessment criteria are defined as follow, according to Tokyo Guidelines 2007 (revised in 2013) (Hirota 2007, Yokoe 2013, Miura 2013):

1. Grade I: Mild acute cholecystitis. There are no findings of organ dysfunctions, and there is mild disease in the gallbladder, allowing for cholecystectomy to be performed as a safe and low-risk procedure. These patients do not have a severity index that meets the criteria for "moderate (Grade II)" or "severe (Grade III)" acute cholecystitis.
2. Grade II: Moderate acute cholecystitis. The degree of acute inflammation is likely to be associated with increased operative difficulty to perform cholecystectomy. Moderate acute cholecystitis is accompanied by any one of the following conditions:
   - Elevated WBC count (>18000/mm^3)
   - Palpable tender mass in the right upper abdominal quadrant
   - Duration of complaints > 72 h (laparoscopic surgery should be performed within 96h after the onset)
   - Marked local inflammation (biliary peritonitis, pericholecystic abscess, hepatic abscess, gangrenous cholecystitis, emphysematous cholecystitis).
3. Grade III: Severe acute Cholecystitis. It is accompanied by dysfuncitions in any one of the following organs/systems:
   - Cardiovascular dysfunction (hypotension requiring treatment with dopamine $\geq$ 5 μg/kg per min, or any dose of dobutamine);
   - Neurological dysfunction (decreased level of consciousness);
   - Respiratory dysfunction (PaO_2/FiO_2 ratio < 300);
   - Renal dysfunction (oliguria, creatinine> 2 mg/dl);
   - Hepatic dysfunction (PT – INR > 1.5);
   - Hematological dysfunction (platelet count < 100000/mm^3).

Differential Diagnosis

Acute cholecystitis could be confused with other causes of sudden pain and tenderness in the right hypochondrium. Acute retrocecal appendicitis, intestinal obstruction, perforated peptic ulcer or acute pancreatitis may produce similar clinical features. Myocardial ischemia, pneumonia, pleuritisand herpes zoster infection involving the intercostal nerves should also be considered.

Severe right upper quadrant pain with high fever and local tenderness may develop in acute gonococcalperihepatitis (Fitz-Hugh-Curtis syndrome).

TREATMENT

Once a patient develops symptoms or complications related to gallstones, such as acute cholecystitis, definitive therapy (cholecystectomy, cholecystostomy, endoscopic sphincterectomy) is recommended in order to avoid the likelihood of subsequent symptoms or complications (Ahmed 2000).

The treatment approach could be as follows:

- Patient with acute cholecystitis should be admitted to the hospital for supportive care, which includes intravenous fluid therapy, correction of electrolyte disorders, and control of pain. Antibiotics should be considered.
- The timing of definitive therapy depends upon the severity of symptoms and the patient overall risk for cholecystectomy.
- If gangrene or perforation are suspected, or if the patient develops progressive symptoms and signs such as fever, hemodynamic instability, or intractable pain while on supportive therapy, emergency cholecystectomy or gallbladder drainage may be needed.
- Low-risk patients without emergent indications for operationgenerally undergo laparoscopic cholecystectomy preferably during the same admission.
- High-risk patients without emergent indications for surgery are treated with a gallbladder drainage procedure if symptoms do not improve with supportive care. For patients whose medical status can be optimized to allow surgery, cholecystectomy can be considered.

Supportive Care

Patient diagnosed with acute calculouscholecystitis have often been ill for days before hospital admission, making intravenous hydration and correction of any associated electrolyte disorders an important initial measure.Patient should be kept fasting.

Pain Control

Pain control can be achieved with nonsteroidal anti-inflammatory drugs (NSAIDs) or opioids. Progression of pain during treatment for acute cholecystitis, despite adequate analgesia, is an indicator of a clinical progression.

Ketorolac (30 to 60 mg), adjusted for age and renal function, given in a single intramuscular dose, usually relieves symptoms of a biliary colic within 20 to 30 minutes.

Patients who can not receive NSAIDs, or who do not achieve adequate pain relief with initial therapy, can be treated with opioids such as morphine or meperidine. It was thought that meperidine was the opioid of choice in patient with gallstone disease because it has less an effect on sphincter of Oddi pressure; however, a systematic review found that all opioids increase sphincter of Oddi pressure and there are insufficient data to suggest that morphine should be avoided.

Antibiotics Acute cholecystitis is primarily an inflammatory process, but secondary infection of the gallbladder may occur. The rate of empyema and pericholecystic abscess is low, but patients can easily develop life-threatening gram negative sepsis from uncomplicated cholecystitis.

Studies are conflicting as to whether antibiotics are required for the treatment of uncomplicated, acute cholecystitis. In fact, the obstruction to bile flow interferes with achieving adequate gallbladder bile concentrations of antibiotics.

Antibiotic therapy should be instituted if sepsis is suspected on the basis of laboratory (WBC count more than 12000/mm^3) or clinical findings (temperature of more than 38.3°C or > 36°C), or in patients with a diagnosis of acute cholecystitis and radiographic findings indicative of gallbladder ischemia or necrosis (i.e., air in the gallbladder or gallbladder wall). Routine antibiotics are also recommended in older patients or those with diabetes or immunodeficiency.

Empiric antibiotic therapy should include activity against the most common pathogens. The most frequent isolates from the gallbladder or common bile duct are Escherichia coli (41%), Enterococcus (12%), Klebsiella (11%), Enterobacter (9%). Thus, broad-spectrum antibiotics should cover gram negative organisms and anaerobes. Commonly used regimens are *piperacillin-tazobactam; ceftriaxone plus metronidazole; levofloxacin plus metronidazole* (Fuks 2013).

Definitive Therapy

The timing and the choice of surgical treatmentfor acute cholecystitis depends upon the severity of symptoms and the patient's overall risk of surgery. The first line treatment of acute cholecystitis is early or urgent cholecystectomy, with laparoscopic cholecystectomy as a preferred method.

Early laparoscopic cholecystectomy is easier to perform, as local inflammation increases 72 hours after the initial onset of symptoms, making dissection less precise, increasing the severity of surgical complications, and making open conversion more likely. In high-risk patients (ASA classes III, IV or V), gallbladder drainage, such as percutaneous transhepatic gallbladder drainage, is an alternative therapy in patients who cannot safely undergo urgent or early cholecystectomy.

Assessment of the operative risk for comorbidities and the patient's general status should also be evaluated in addition to the severity grade of cholecystitis.

1. Grade I (mild) acute cholecystitis: early laparoscopic cholecystectomy is the first line treatment.
2. Grade II (moderate) acute cholecystitis: elective cholecystectomy after the improvement of the acute inflammatory process is the first-line treatment. If a patient does not respond to initial medical treatment, urgent or early gallbladder drainage is required. Grade II acute cholecystitis with serious local complications is an indication for urgent cholecystectomy and drainage.
3. Grade III (severe) acute cholecystitis: appropriate organ support such as ventilatory/circulatory management in addition to initial medical treatment is necessary. Urgent or early gallbladder drainage should be performed. Elective cholecystectomy may be performed after the improvement of acute illness has been achieved by gallbladder drainage.

Surgical Approach

Laparoscopic cholecystectomy is considered the standard approach for the surgical treatment of acute calculouscholecystitis (Gurusamy 2013). Compared with open cholecystectomy, laparoscopic cholecystectomy reduces postoperative pain and significantly shortens hospital length of stay and convalescence, and time away from work. However, the overall serious complication rate in laparoscopic approach remains higher than that seen with open surgery (Brooks 2013, Wu 2015, Yamashita 2007).

Other techniques such as single-incision laparoscopy, mini-laparoscopy, robotic-assisted laparoscopy, and natural orifice transuminal endoscopic surgery (NOTES) have been used to treat patients with cholelithiasis, but their role in the treatment of acute cholecystitis is limited, due to the technically demanding dissection caused by severe inflammation (Reis 1990).

For patients in whom the risk for injury or excessive blood loss is deemed too high to perform cholecystectomy, a cholecystostomy or a subtotal cholecystectomy can be performed. The latter procedure achieves control of the cystic duct at the level of the neck of the gallbladder and leaves the dome of the gallbladder adherent to the liver fossa in situ. Biliary leaks may occur, but it can be managed conservatively.

Gallbladder Drainage

Gallbladder drainage is required for high-risk patients managed conservatively but who show no appreciable improvement and progress to severe symptoms. The aim of the drainage is to direct purulent material away from the obstructed gallbladder, which also allows for resolution of edema, which often opens up the obstructed cystic duct.

Gallbladder drainage can be accomplished via percutaneous, endoscopic, or surgical approaches.

- *Percutaneous* – it is indicated for patients with acute cholecystitis who have contraindications to general anesthesia; severe cholecystitis; late presentation (>72 hours after onset of symptoms); failure of medical (antibiotic) therapy. Percutaneous cholecystostomy resolves acute cholecystitis in approximately 90% of patients (Figure 4). Decompressing the gallbladder allows both local inflammation and systemic illness to resolve, before gallbladder removal could be accomplished with less risk to the patient. The timing of cholecystectomy after gallbladder drainage can be variable, ranging from immediately after clinical improvement to after eight weeks.

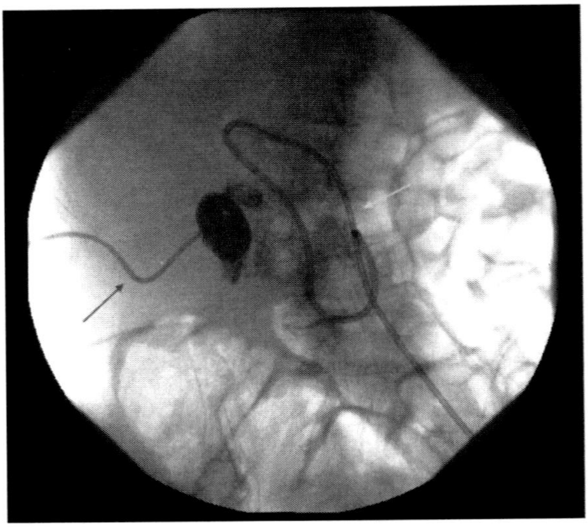

Figure 4. X-ray of the abdomen showing a percutaneous cholecystostomy performed with a 10F catheter (red arrow) in a patient with obstructive jaundice previously treated with percutaneous biliary drainage (yellowarrow).

Minor complications of percutaneous drainage include bleeding, catheter blockage and dislodgement, and failure to resolve the acute cholecystitis (10%).Failure is usually related to ineffective drainage due to thick sludge or pus; it is possible to irrigate the gallbladder contents manually with normal saline solution through the catheter but if irrigation is ineffective, the percutaneous pigtail catheter can be replaced with a larger one to achieve more effective irrigation (Akhan 2002, Joseph 2012, Spira 2002).

Percutaneous cholecystostomy is often performed with the intent of delayed cholecystectomy; patients who stabilize but continue to be high risk for surgery can be considered for percutaneous gallstone extraction with or without mechanical litotripsy (Cherng 2012, Simorov 2013).

- *Endoscopic* - Endoscopic gallbladder drainage can be performed in patients with acute cholecystitis in whom percutaneous approaches are contraindicated, or are not anatomically feasible (i.e., advanced liver disease, ascites, coagulopathy). Two different techinques are available: transpapillary drainage or transmural drainage (Kjaer 2007).

- *Transpapillary drainage*It utilizes endoscopic retrograde cholangiography (ERCP) techniques and equipment to place a drainage catheter into the gallbladder via the cystic duct. The other end of the catheter is brought out through the nose (naso-biliary drain) or left to drain internally into the duodenum. Transpapillary drainage resolves acute cholecystectomy in 80 to 90% of patients, including those with advanced liver cirrhosis. This technique can be technically challenging because the cystic duct is often narrow and tortuous.
- *Transmural drainage*It utilizes endoscopic ultrasound guidance to access the inflamed gallbladder with a needle puncture, followed by dilation and stent placement over a guidewire. The introduction of self-expandable, covered, lumen-apposing metal stents allows direct endoscopic access to the gallbladder for decompression and stone removal. The transmural drainage resolves acute cholecystitis in over 95% of patients. Endoscopic transmural drainage is used as a bridge to definitive gallbladder surgery; however, the adhesion created between the gallbladder and duodenum/stomach may interfere with future cholecystectomy surgery.

- *Surgical* Although high-risk patients are generally treated with antibiotic therapy with or without a gallbladder drainage procedure, an initial surgical approach may be preferred in some patients for whom the burden of the ongoing systemic effects of cholecystitis is deemed to be greater than the risk of surgery. If medical risk precludes gallbladder removal, a surgical cholecystostomy tube can be inserted through a limited laparotomy.

For patients who undergo gallbladder drainage, the subsequent care depends on whether clinical symptoms resolve after the procedure.

Patients who have become reasonable candidates for surgery should undergo elective cholecystectomy.

If the less-invasive techniques are not technically feasible, are unsuccessful at providing adequate drainage, or if the patient does not improve following drainage, a surgical approach may become necessary. Laparoscopic cholecystectomy is preferred.

COMPLICATIONS

The major complications of acute cholecystitis are empyema, gangrene and perforation.

Empyema

If the cystic duct remains blocked by a stone and infection sets in, empyema may develop. In this case, the gallbladder contains frank pus; symptoms may be of an intra-abdominal abscess with high spiking fever (39°-40°), chills, and leukocytosis greater than 15.000/μl. Parenteral antibiotics should be given, and percutaneous cholecystostomy or cholecystectomy should be performed.

Gangrene

Gangrenous cholecystitis is the most common complication of cholecystitis, particularly in older patients, diabetic patients, or those who delay seeking therapy. The presence of a sepsis-like picture in addition to the other symptoms of cholecystitis suggests the diagnosis, but gangrene may not be suspected preoperatively.

Perforation

Acute calcolouscholecystitis may proceed to complete necrosis of the gallbladder wall and perforation. The gallstone may erode the necrotic wall; alternatively, dilated infected Rokitansky-Aschoff sinuses may provide a weak point for rupture. Rupture usually takes place at the fundus which is the least well-vascularized part of the gallbladder. Rupture into the free peritoneal cavity is rare and, more usually, adhesions form between adjacent organs with local abscess formation. Rupture into adjacent viscera leads to internal biliary fistula. The patient presents with nausea, right upper quadrant pain and vomiting. A right upper quadrant mass is palpable in 50%, and a similar number are febrile. The diagnosis is often overlooked. CT and US are of value in showing peritoneal fluid, abscess and gallstones (Roslyn 1987). There are three clinical types:

1. *Acute with bile peritonitis.* It is often associated with systemic conditions including vascular insufficiency or immunodeficiency such as atherosclerosis, diabetes mellitus, collagen diseases, corticosteroid use or decompensated cirrhosis. Prognosis is poor with a mortality of about 30%. Treatment is by massive antibiotics and restoration of the fluid balance. The gangrenous gallbladder wall is removed or drained percutaneously or surgically. Any abscess must also be drained (Figure 5).
2. *Subacute with pericholecystic abscess.* These patients have chronic gallstone disease and the picture is intermediate between the acute and chronic types.
3. *Chronic* with cholecystenteric fistula formation. Fistulas are usually asymptomatic, unless the gallbladder is still partially obstructed by stones. If the gallbladder stones discharge through the fistula and if they are large enough, they may obstruct the small intestine (gallstone ileus) (Figure 6).

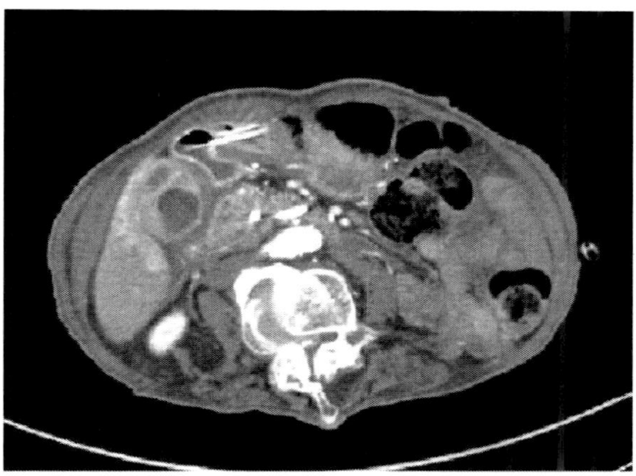

Figure 5.Computed tomography of the abdomen showing agallbladder with Thickened wall and pericholecystic abscess (contained perforation)in a patient with acute calculouscholecystitis.

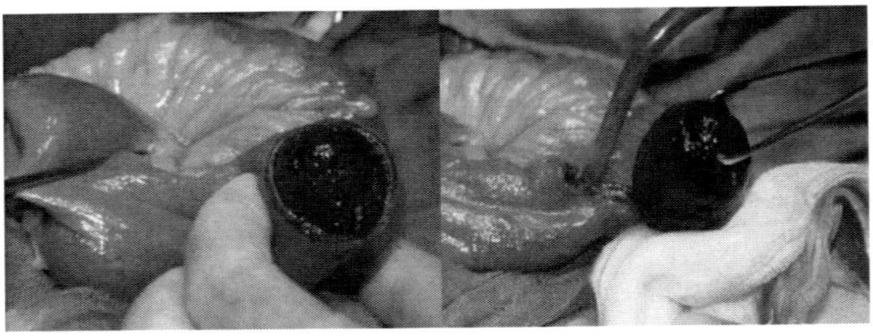

Figure 6. Intraoperative small bowel extraction of gallstone in a patient with intestinal obstruction (gallstone ileus).

Emphysematous Cholecystitis

Emphysematous cholecystitis is caused by secondary infection of the gallbladder wall with gas-forming organisms (such as Clostridium welchii). Other organisms that may be isolated include Escherichia coli (15 per cent), staphylococci, streptococci, Pseudomonas and Klebsiella.

Affected patients are often men in their fifth to seventh decade, and approximately one-third to one-half have diabetes. Gallstones are present in about one-half of patients.

Patients usually present with right upper quadrant pain, nausea, vomiting and low-grade fever. Peritoneal signs are usually absent but crepitus in the abdominal wall adjacent to the gallbladder may rarely be detected. When such crepitus is present, it is an important clue to the diagnosis. Mild to moderate unconjugated hyperbilirubinemia may be present, caused by hemolysis induced by clostridial infection. The ultrasound report may erroneously note "overlying bowel gas making adequate visualization of the gallbladder difficult", when in reality this reflects air in the wall of the gallbladder. Emphysematous cholecystitis often heralds the development of gangrene and perforation (Lorenz 1990).

Acalculous Cholecystitis

Acalculous Cholecystitis is an acute inflammatory disease of the gallbladder with a multifactorial pathogenesis. It accounts for approximately 10% of all cases of acute cholecystitis and is associated with high morbidity and mortality rates.

Pathogenesis

Acalculous Cholecystitis is typically seen in patients who are hospitalized and critically ill. Bile stasis is considered the primary etiologic factor which results in increased mucosal susceptibility to injury. Systemic bacterial or fungal infection then colonizes the static bile in the biliary tree, providing a medium for bacterial growth. Ischemic mucosal injury is also thought to play an etiological role. A history of hypotensive episodes and atherosclerotic disease is frequently present in patients who develop acute Acalculous Cholecystitis. Beltrame et al. (2012) described a case of a 29-year-old female with acute Acalculous Cholecystitis associated with EBV infection. The patient was successfully treated with conservative therapy.

Diagnosis

In these patients, the appearance of unexplained fever, leukocytosis, or vague abdominal discomfort may be the only signs of Acalculous Cholecystitis. Patients may also have jaundice or a right upper quadrant mass. Laboratory test abnormalities may include a leukocytosis or abnormal liver test, but they are non-specific. Gallbladder necrosis, gangrene, and perforation could be present at the time of diagnosis. These complications may result in sepsis, shock and peritonitis.

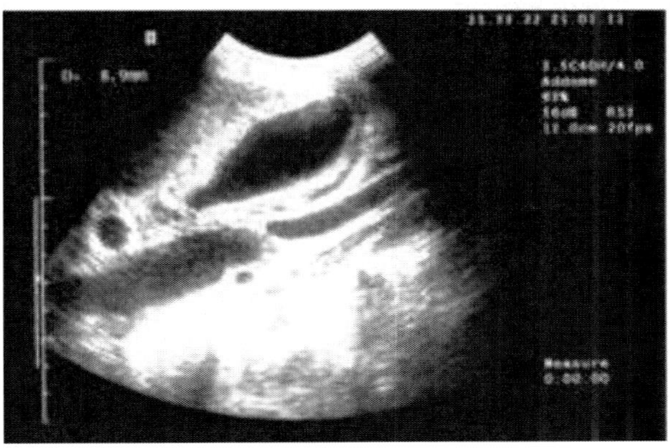

Figure 7.Ultrasonography of the abdomen showing an enlarged gallbladder with thickened wall and pericholecistic fluid (acute Acalculous Cholecystitis).

Imaging

Ultrasonography is typically the first test when Acalculous Cholecystitis is suspected. US has good sensitivity and specificity for diagnosing Acalculous Cholecystitis.

Treatment

Initiation of broad spectrum antibiotics is recommended. Infection with enteric pathogens, including *E.coli, E. faecalis, Klebsiella, Pseudomonas, Proteus* species, and *Bacteroides* is common, and antibiotics should cover these organisms. Vancomycin can be added if nosocomial infection with methicillin-resistant Staphylococcus aureus (MRSA) is known or suspected.

Cholecystectomy or cholecystostomy is recommended rather than supportive care; prompt treatment is imperative, because gallbladder gangrene may develop and can result in gallbladder perforation. Untreated Acalculous Cholecystitis is associated with mortality rates of up to 70%. Cholecystostomy is less invasive, however, cholecystectomy should be performed if there are findings suggesting gallbladder necrosis, emphysematous cholecystitis, or perforation.

Patients who fail to improve or worsen following cholecystostomy require cholecystectomy. Failure to improve may be due to gangrenous cholecystitis, catheter dislodgement, bile leakage resulting in peritonitis, or an incorrect diagnosis (McChesney 2003, Wang 2003, Ryu 2003).

References

Ahmed, A., Cheung, R.C. and Keeffe, E.B. (2000). Management of gallstones and their complications. *Am. Fam. Physician*,*61*,1673-80, 1687-8.

Akhan, O., Akinci, D. and Ozmen, M.N. (2002). Percutaneous cholecystostomy. *Eur. J. Radiol.*,*43*, 229-36.

Beltrame, V., Andres, A. L., Tona, F. and Sperti, C. (2012). Epstein-Barr virus – associate acute Acalculous Cholecystitis in an adult. *Am. J. Case Rep.*, *13*, 153-156.

Bree, R.L. (1995). Further observations on the usefulness of the sonographic Murphy sign in the evaluation of suspected acute cholecystitis. *J. Clin. Ultrasound*,*23*, 169–72.

Brooks, K. R., Scarborough, J.E., Vaslef, S.N. and Shapiro, M.L. (2013). No need to wait: an analysis of the timing of cholecystectomy during admission for acute cholecystitis using the American College of Surgeons National Surgical Quality Improvement Program database. *J. Trauma Acute Care Surg.*, *74*, 167-73, 173-4.

Chatziioannou, S.N., Moore, W.H., Ford, P.V. and Dhekne, R. D. (2000). Hepatobiliary scintigraphy is superior to abdominal ultrasonography in suspected acute cholecystitis. *Surgery,127*, 609-13.

Cherng, N., Witkowski, E.T., Sneider, E.B., et al., (2012). Use of cholecystostomy tubes in the management of patients with primary diagnosis of acute cholecystitis. *J. Am. Coll. Surg.,214*, 196-201.

Cooperberg, P.L. and Burhenne, H.J. (1980). Real-time ultrasonography. Diagnostic technique of choice in calculous gallbladder disease. *N. Engl. J. Med.,302*, 1277-9.

Fidler, J., Paulson, E.K. and Layfield, L. (1996). CT evaluation of acute cholecystitis: findings and usefulness in diagnosis.*Am. J. Roentgenol.,166*, 1085-8.

Friedman, G.D. (1993). Natural history of asymptomatic and symptomatic gallstones. *Am. J. Surg.,165*,399-404.

Fuks, D., Cossé, C. and Régimbeau, J.M., (2013). Antibiotic therapy in acute calculous cholecystitis. *J. Visc. Surg.,150*, 3-8

Gurusamy, K.S., Davidson, C., Gluud, C. and Davidson, B.R. (2013). Early versus delayed laparoscopic cholecystectomy for people with acute cholecystitis. *Cochrane DatabaseSyst. Rev.,6*, CD005440.

Hafif, A., Gutman, M., Kaplan, O., Winkler, E., Rozin, R.R. and Skornick, Y. (1991). The management of acute cholecystitis in elderly patients. *Am. Surg.,57*, 648–52.

Hirota, M., Takada, T., Kawarada, Y., Nimura, Y., Miura, F., Hirata, K., et al , (2007). Diagnostic criteria and severity assessment of acute cholecystitis: Tokyo Guidelines. *J. HepatobiliaryPancreat. Surg.,14*, 78–82.

Indar, A. and Beckingham, I. (2002). Acute cholecystitis. *B.M.J.,325*, 639–43

Johannsen, E. C. and Madoff, L. C. (2005). Infections of the liver and biliary system. In: Mandell GL, Bennett JE, Dolin R, editors. *Principles of practice of infectious diseases*. Philadelphia: Elsevier, 951–8.

Joseph, T., Unver, K., Hwang, G.L., et al., (2012). Percutaneous cholecystostomy for acute cholecystitis: ten-yearexperience. *J. Vasc. Interv. Radiol.23*, 83-8.

Juvonen, T., Kiviniemi, H., Niemela, O. and Kairaluoma, M. I. (1992). Diagnostic accuracy of ultrasonography and C reactive protein concentration in acute cholecystitis: a prospective clinical study. *Eur. J. Surg.,158*, 365-9.

Kalimi, R., Gecelter, G.R., Caplin, D., et al., (2001). Diagnosis of acute cholecystitis: sensitivity of sonography, cholescintigraphy, and combined sonography-cholescintigraphy. *J. Am. Coll. Surg,193*, 609-613.

Kaminski, D.L. (1989). Arachidonic acid metabolites in hepatobiliary physiology and disease. *Gastroenterology,97*, 781-92.

Kiewiet, J.J., Leeuwenburgh, M.M., Bipat, S., et al., (2012). A systematic review and meta-analysis of diagnostic performance of imaging in acute cholecystitis. *Radiology,264*, 708-20.

Kjaer, D.W., Kruse, A. and Funch-Jensen, P. (2007). Endoscopic gallbladder drainage of patients with acute cholecystitis. *Endoscopy,39*, 304-8.

Lillemoe, K.D. (2000). Surgical treatment of biliary tract infections. *Am. Surg.,66*, 138–44.

Lorenz, R.W. and Steffen, H.M. (1990). Emphysematous cholecystitis: diagnostic problems and differential diagnosis of gallbladder gas accumulations. *Hepatogastroenterology,37*Suppl 2, 103-6.

Martinez, A., Bona, X., Velasco, M. and Martin, J. (1986). Diagnostic accuracy of ultrasound in acute cholecystitis. *Gastrointest. Radiol.11*, 334–8.

McChesney, J.A., Northup, P.G. and Bickston, S.J. (2003). Acute acalculous cholecystitis associated with systemic sepsis and visceral arterial hypoperfusion: a case series and review of patophysiology. *Dig. Dis. Sci.,48*, 1960-7.

Miura, F., Takada, T., Strasberg, S.M., et al., (2013). TG13 flow chart for the management of acute cholangitis and cholecystitis. *J. Hepatobiliary Pancreat. Surg.,20*, 47-54.

Ralls, P.W., Coletti, P.M., Halls, J.M., et al. (1982). Prospective evaluation of 99m TC-IDA cholescintigraphy in the diagnosis of acute cholecystitis. *Radiology,144*, 369–71.

Ralls, P.W., Halls, J., Lapin, S.A., Quinn, M.F., Morris, U.L. and Boswell, W. (1982). Prospective evaluation of the sonographic Murphy sign in suspected acute cholecystitis. *J. Clin. Ultrasound,10*, 113–5.

Ralls, P.W., Colletti, P.M., Lapin, S.A., et al., (1985). Real-time sonography in suspected acute cholecystitis. Prospective evaluation of primary and secondary signs. *Radiology,155*, 767-71.

Reiss, R., Nudelman, I., Gutman, C. and Deutsch, A. A. (1990). Changing trends in surgery for acute cholecystitis. *World. J. Surg.*,*14*, 567-70.

Roslyn, J.J., DenBesten, L., Thompson, J.E. Jr, and Silverman, B.F. (1980). Roles of lithogenic bile and cystic duct occlusion in the pathogenesis of acute cholecystitis. *Am. J. Surg.*,*140*, 126-30.

Roslyn, J.J., Thompson, J.E. Jr, Darvin, H. and DenBesten, L. (1987). Risk factors for gallbladder perforation. *Am. J. Gastroenterol.*,*82*, 636-40.

Ryu, J.K., Ryu, K.H. and Kim, K.H. (2003). Clinical features of acute acalculous cholecystitis. *J. Clin. Gastroenterol.*,*36*, 166-9.

Shapiro, M.J., Luchtefeld, W.B., Kurzweil, S., Kaminski, D.L., Durham, R.M. and Mazuski, J.E. (1994). Acute acalculous cholecystitis in the critically ill. *Am. Surg.*,*60*, 335–9.

Shea, J.A., Berlin, J.A., Escarce, J.J., Clarke, J.R., Kinosian, B.P., Cabana, M.D., et al., (1994). Revised estimates of diagnostic test sensitivity and specificity in suspected biliary tract disease. *Arch. Intern. Med.*,*154*, 2573-81.

Simorov, A., Ranade, A., Parcells, J., et al., (2013). Emergent cholecystostomy is superior to open cholecystectomy in extremely ill patients with a calculous cholecystitis; a large multi center out come study. *Am. J. Surg.*,*206*, 935-40.

Singer, A.J., McCracken, G., Henry, M.C., et al. (1996). Correlation among clinical, laboratory and hepatobiliary scanning findings in patients with suspected acute cholecystitis. *Ann. Emerg. Med.*,*28*,267-72.

Spira, R.M., Nissan, A., Zamir, O., et al., (2002). Percutaneous transhepaticcholecystostomy and delayed laparoscopiccholecystectomy in critically ill patients with acute calculous cholecystitis. *Am. J. Surg.*, 2002,*183*, 62-6.

Steven, M. and Strasberg, M.D. (2008). Acute calculous cholecystitis. *N. Engl. J. Med.*,*358*, 2804-11.

Trowbridge, R.L., Rutkowski, N.K. and Shojania, K.G. (2003). Does this patient have acute cholecystitis? *JAMA*,*289*, 80-6.

Wang, A.J., Wang, T.E., Lin, C.C., et al., (2003). Clinical predictors of severe gallbladder complications in acute acalculous cholecystitis. *World. J. Gastroenterol.*,*9*, 2821-3.

Wu, X.D., Tian, X., Liu, M.M., et al., (2015). Meta-analysis comparing early versus delayed laparoscopiccholecystectomy for acute cholecystitis. *Br. J. Surg.,102*, 1302-13.

Yamashita, Y., Takada, T., Kawarada, Y., et al., (2007). Surgical treatment of patients with acute cholecystitis: Tokyo Guidelines. *J. Hepatobiliary Pancreat. Surg.,14*, 91-7.

Yokoe, M., Takada, T., Strasberg, S.M., et al., (2013). TG13 diagnostic criteria and severity grading of acute cholecystitis. *J. Hepatobiliary Pancreat. Surg.,20*, 35-46.

In: Acute Cholecystitis
Editor: Lisa Powell

ISBN: 978-1-63485-744-4

Chapter 2

DIAGNOSIS AND TREATMENT OF ACUTE CHOLECYSTITIS

María Cristina Nevado García, Jaime Ruiz-Tovar Polo, David Alias Jiménez, Pedro Yuste and Eduardo Ferrero Herrero
General surgery, Madrid, Spain

ABSTRACT

Acute cholecystitis is a common emergency presentation of gallstone disease. The improvements in diagnosis and treatment can lead to reduce rates of morbidity, mortality and costs.

Clinical findings are usually diagnostic of acute cholecystitis. However, imaging studies play an important role in the confirmation of the diagnosis and detection of associated complications.

On physical examination patients typically present severe right upper quadrant pain with positive Murphy sign associated with nausea, vomits and fever. Leukocytosis with neutrophilia is the most common laboratory finding, while elevated liver enzymes are related with worse outcome.

Imaging studies allow clinicians to establish diagnosis in suspected individuals and to detect complications. Right upper quadrant ultrasound is the imaging modality of choice due to its sensitivity (82%), specificity (81%), availability, low cost and lack of radiation exposure. Computed Tomography (CT) is currently recommended when other intraabdominal pathologies are suspected and Magnetic Resonance Imaging (MRI) is useful for pregnant patients and to identify choledocholithiasis.

Once the diagnosis of acute cholecystitis is achieved, we must take decisions in order to provide patients the best management available. Despite of overtime controverses about the optimal treatment, early laparoscopic cholecystectomy is currently accepted as the best option. Surgery should be performed as soon as possible after diagnosis, because it reduces total hospital stay and does not increase complication or conversion rates. Percutaneous cholecystostomy is indicated in the advanced form of inflammation or in patients with severe comorbidities increasing surgical risk.

INTRODUCTION

The term *cholecystitis* defines an inflammation of the gallbladder. Although most people with gallstones do not have symptoms and will not go on to develop cholecystitis, cholecystitis occurs most commonly due to blockage of the cystic duct with gallstones (cholelithiasis). This blockage causes a buildup of bile in the gallbladder and increased pressure within the gallbladder, leading to right upper abdominal pain. Concentrated bile, pressure, and sometimes bacterial infection irritate and damage the gallbladder wall, causing inflammation and swelling of the gallbladder, which might reduce normal blood flow to areas of the gallbladder, leading to necrosis due to inadequate oxygenation.

Risk factors for gallstones and cholecystitis are similar and include female sex, increasing age, pregnancy, oral contraceptives, obesity, diabetes mellitus and rapid weight loss (including postoperative course of bariatric surgery) [1].

Acute cholecystitis is a common emergency presentation of gallstone disease. Recent improvements in diagnosis and treatment can lead to reduce rates of morbidity, mortality and costs.

DIAGNOSIS

Clinical findings are usually diagnostic for acute cholecystitis. Severe, steady and prolonged right upper quadrant pain with associated fever, nausea, vomiting and anorexia are the most common symptoms.

On physical examination patients typically appear ill, with voluntary and involuntary abdominal guarding and with a positive Murphy´s sign that is usually diagnostic for acute cholecystitis. To check for a Murphy's sign, the patient is asked to inspire deeply while the examiner palpates the area of the gallbladder fossa just beneath the liver edge. Deep inspiration causes the gallbladder to descend and press against the examining fingers, which in patients with acute cholecystitis commonly leads to increased discomfort and the patient stopping the breath. General patient conditions are related with time elapsed since the beginning of the clinical manifestations [2].

Patients with complications may have signs of sepsis (gangrene), generalized peritonitis (perforation), abdominal crepitus (emphysematous cholecystitis), or bowel obstruction (gallstone ileus).

Nevertheless, it must be considered that there is a variable clinical presentation that depends on the underlying patient conditions, comorbidities and time of clinical evolution.

In the laboratory data, patients typically have leukocytosis with an increased number of band forms. Elevation in the serum total bilirubin and alkaline phosphatase concentrations are not common in uncomplicated acute cholecystitis, as biliary obstruction is limited to the gallbladder. When present, it should raise concerns about complicating conditions such as cholangitis, choledocholithiasis, or Mirizzi syndrome (a gallstone impacted in the distal cystic duct causing extrinsic compression of the common bile duct) [3].

However, there have been reports of mild elevations in serum aminotransferases and amylase, along with hyperbilirubinemia and jaundice, even in the absence of these complications. These abnormalities may be due to the passage of small stones, sludge, or pus.

Even though the combination of history, clinical signs, laboratory values and physical examination are usually diagnostic for acute cholecystitis, imaging findings play an important role in the confirmation of the diagnosis and detection of associated complications [4].

Among the multiple imaging modalities that are available for the diagnosis of acute cholecystitis, both clinicians and radiologist should be aware of the advantages and drawbacks of each technique in order to select the most appropriate study tailored to the needs of the patient.

Abdominal ultrasound is the imaging modality of choice in suspected cases of acute cholecystitis, due to low cost, availability and lack of radiation exposure. It is a fast and safe technique with a sensitivity and specificity values of 82% and 81% respectively for the diagnosis of acute cholecystitis. Sonographic features that lead us to the diagnosis are:

- Cholelitiasis
- Gallbladder wall thickening (greater than 4 to 5 mm) or edema (double wall sign) is the most reliable diagnostic feature

- A “sonographic Murphy’s sign” is similar to the Murphy’s sign elicited during abdominal examination, except that the positive response is observed during palpation with the ultrasound transducer. This is more accurate than hand palpation, because it can confirm that it is indeed the gallbladder that is being pressed by the imaging transducer when the patient catches the breath.
- Pericholecystic fluid

The gallbladder may be decompressed in perforated cases and there will be associated pericholecystic or perihepatic fluid collections as well as we can find gas bubbles in emphysematous cholecystitis [5].

Another imaging technique with diagnostic accuracy values comparable to ultrasound is the magnetic resonance (MR). It is helpful in the detection of common bile duct stones and allows the definition of pancreatic and biliary tract anatomy. Despite its good diagnostic performance, the availability, cost and time required for the exploration, limit its use in the diagnosis of acute cholecystitis. However, MR is indicated in patients with suspected biliary obstruction secondary to choledocholithiasis and in pregnant patients with right upper quadrant abdominal pain [6].

Computed tomography (CT) is not included in the first line diagnostic techniques. It is less sensitive and specific in the diagnosis of cholecystitis (73% and 42-74% respectively). CT scan is recommended when other intraabdominal pathology is suspected, in cases of uncertain diagnosis and is particulary useful to detect complications such as perforation, hemorrhage, emphysema and abscess formation. CT findings include cholelithiasis, gallbladder distention, mural or mucosal hyperenhancement, wall thickening and edema and pericholecystic fluid [7].

There are another diagnosis techniques described in the literature as Hepatobiliary iminodiacetic acid scan (HIDA) or endoscopic ultrasound. This procedures are reserved for cases with unclear diagnosis.

TREATMENT

Once the diagnosis of acute cholecystitis is achieved, we must take decisions in order to provide patients the best management available.

The first measure is the supportive care: intravenous hydration and correction of any associated electrolyte disorders, pain control and antibiotics.

Nonesteroidal antiinflammatory drugs are the first line drugs used. Opioids are also aceptable alternatives for acute pain. Antimicrobial therapy is administered to all patients diagnosed with acute cholecystitis, which are continued until the gallbladder is removed or the cholecystitis clinically resolves. When antibiotic therapy is initiated, the duration of postoperative treatment is generally tailored to the clinical situation. Empiric antibiotic therapy should include activity against the most common pathogens. The most frequent isolates from the gallbladder or common bile duct were Escherichia coli, followed by Enterococcus spp, Klebsiella spp and Enterobacter spp. Thus, broad-spectrum antibiotics should cover gram-negative organisms and anaerobes. Commonly used regimens are piperacillin-tazobactam, ceftriaxone plus metronidazole, or levofloxacin plus metronidazole. Antibiotic therapy should subsequently be tailored to culture and susceptibility results when available [8].

The next step is the definitive therapy. The selection and timing of this therapy depends upon the severity of symptoms and the patient's overall risk for cholecystectomy [9].

As we can see in Figure 1, patients with high operative risk should be candidates to conservative management (intravenous fluids and antibiotics). In these cases, when the clinical situation is not improving, a percutaneous cholecystostomy should be indicated. This technique allows an image-guided gallbladder drainage. It can be performed through a transhepatic or transperitoneal approach, although the transhepatic is preferred due to a greater stability of the catheter, lower risk of bile peritonitis and bowel injury [10].

However, in operable candidates with acute cholecystitis, a cholecystectomy with intravenous antibiotics is the treatment of choice.

Since the development of laparoscopic procedures the timing of cholecystectomy for acute cholecystitis became controversial. The learning curve of laparoscopic cholecystectomy, the conversion rates to open cholecystectomy and the risk of bile duct injuries during the acute phase were the principal drawbacks for this surgical technique against the conservative management with antibiotics and delayed cholecystectomy [2].

Several studies analyzed the risk of conversion and operative injuries, costs, total hospital stay, morbidity and mortality rates. One of the most recent reviews, in 2013, including five randomized controlled trials with 451 patients, compared early (within 7 days of presentation) to late (> 6 weeks after presentation) laparoscopic cholecystectomy for acute cholecystitis. No differences in postoperative infection, bile duct injury or conversion to open cholecystectomy were demonstrated between patients undergoing early versus late cholecystectomy. The benefit towards early performance was in costs, total hospital stay and number of readmissions [11].

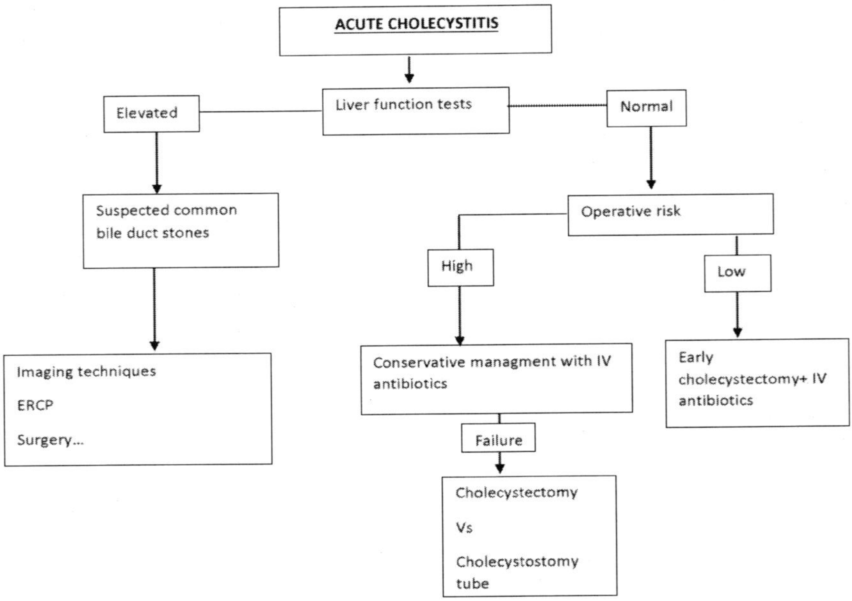

Figure 1. Treatment for acute cholecystitis.

The evidence available in the literature supports the recommendation about laparoscopic cholecystectomy as the treatment of choice for acute cholecystitis and surgery should be performed as soon as possible after the diagnosis. Open conversion may be necessary and should not be considered a failure in management. Cholecystectomy during index admission is associated with decreased in-hospital mortality, long-term mortality and gallstone-related readmission. In those patients who do not undergo cholecystectomy during initial hospitalization experience, recurrence rates of gallstone complications range from 20 to 50% [12].

However, this is a very heterogeneous disease with general and local factors that must be considered. This could present with a picture ranging from mild, self-limiting, to a potentially life-threatening illness. The condition of the patient with their comorbidities and the degree of gallbladder inflammation are decisive to indicate the best therapeutic option for every single patient.

REFERENCES

[1] Strasberg SM. Clinical practice. Acute calculous cholecystitis. N. Eng. J Med. 2008; 358: 2804–11.

[2] Duncan CB, Riall TS. Evidence-based current surgical practice: calculous gallbladder disease. J Gastrointest Surg 2012; 16: 2011-2025.

[3] Knab LM, Boller AM, Mahvi DM. Cholecystitis. Surg. Clin. North Am. 2014; 94: 455-470.

[4] Kiewiet JJ, Leeuwenburgh MM, Bipat S, et al. A systematic review and meta-analysis of diagnostic performance of imaging in acute cholecystitis. Radiology 2012; 264: 708-720.

[5] Katabathina VS, Zafar AM, Suri R. Clinical presentation, imaging, and management of acute cholecystitis. Tech. Vasc. Interventional Rad. 2015; 18: 256-265.

[6] Tonolini M, Ravelli A, Villa C, et al. Urgent MRI with MR colangiopancreatography (MRCP) of acute cholecystitis and related complications: diagnostic role and spectrum of imaging findings. Emerg. Radiol. 2012; 19: 341-348.

[7] Patel NB, Oto A, Thomas S. Multidetector CT of emergent biliary pathologic conditions. Radiographics 2013; 33: 1867-1888.

[8] Mazeh H, Mizrahi I, Dior U, et al. Role of antibiotic therapy in mild acute calculus cholecystitis: A prospective randomized controlled trial. World J. Surg. 2012; 36:1750.

[9] Ambe PC, Papadakis M, Zirngibl H. A proposal for a preoperative clinical scoring system for acute cholecystitis. J. Surg. Res. 2016; 200: 473-479.

[10] Campanile FC, Pisano M, Coccolini F, et al. Acute cholecystitis: WSES position statement. World J. Emerg. Surg. 2014; 9:58.

[11] Gurusamy KS, Davidson C, Gluud C, et al. Early versus delayed laparoscopic cholecystectomy for people with acute cholecystitis. Cochrane Database Syst. Rev. 2013; 6: :CD005440.

[12] Cao AM, Eslick GD, Cox MR. Early laparoscopic cholecystectomy is superior to delayed acute cholecystitis: a meta-analysis of case-control studies. Surg. Endosc. 2015; DOI 10.10007/s00464-015-4325-4.

In: Acute Cholecystitis
Editor: Lisa Powell

ISBN: 978-1-63485-744-4

Chapter 3

DIAGNOSTIC WORK-UP OF PATIENTS WITH ACUTE CHOLECYSTITIS

Andrei M. Beliaev[1,*]***, Michael Booth***[2,†]***, Neville Angelo***[3,‡] ***and Colleen Bergin***[4,§]

[1]Green Lane Cardiothoracic Surgical Unit,
Auckland City Hospital, Auckland, New Zealand
[2]Department of General Surgery, North Shore Hospital,
Auckland, New Zealand
[3]Department of Pathology, North Shore Hospital,
Auckland, New Zealand
[4]Department of of Radiology, Auckland City Hospital,
Auckland, New Zealand

ABSTRACT

Introduction: The diagnosis of acute cholecystitis (AC) can be challenging, may result in misdiagnosis, patient's hospital discharge without operation, delay in cholecystectomy and increased mortality. To improve accuracy in the diagnosis of AC, the 2007 and 2013 Tokyo

* Address for correspondence and reprints: Dr Andrei M. Beliaev; Cardiothoracic Surgical Unit, Auckland City Hospital, Private Bag 92024, Auckland, New Zealand; Tel (09) 307 4949 ext 22787; Fax (09) 307 4944; Email: AndreiB@adhb.govt.nz.

† Michael.Booth@waitematadhb.govt.nz.

‡ Neville.Angello@waitematadhb.govt.nz.

§ Colleen.Bergin@adhb.govt.nz.

guidelines (TG07/TG13) added elevated concentration of C-reactive protein (CRP) as one of the analytic criteria. However, CRP is not widely used for diagnosing AC and its grade of severity. To determine the utility of CRP in the diagnosis of AC, the discriminative power of CRP was compared with that of white cell count (WCC) in patients with AC of different histological grades of severity. We found that CRP had a better discriminative power than WCC in predicting the histological severity of AC including acute on chronic, acute edematous, necrotizing, suppurative and gangrenous cholecystitis. We suggest that leucopenia (WCC < $4000/mm^3$) and combinations of systemic signs of inflammation should be added to modify the Tokyo diagnostic criteria for AC. Patients with acute on chronic and acute edematous cholecystitis had low rates of CTO and were therefore included in the mild category of AC. Patients with acute necrotizing, suppurative, gangrenous cholecystitis, pericholecystic abscess and AC with gallbladder perforation were allocated to the moderate - severe category of AC and these were associated with a twofold increased risk of CTO.

Conclusion: Tokyo diagnostic criteria for AC should be modified to include combinations of more than one systemic sign of inflammation as indicators of severity, and, leucopenia should be added as an analytic criterion.

1.0. INTRODUCTION

The prevalence of gallstones in an adult Western community lies between 15% and 20% [1, 2]. In the United States, an estimated 11.8 million individuals aged between 20 and 74 years have cholelithiasis [3]. Each year approximately 1% to 2% of people with silent gallstones develop symptoms and are admitted to a hospital for treatment [4-6]. Of these, 20% present with acute cholecystitis (AC), which in the elderly and patients with significant co-morbidities is associated with a 2% - 3% mortality [5, 7, 8]. In 2009 cholecystitis was reported as the underlying cause of death in more than 2000 patients in the United States, and a contributing cause of death in about 3300 patients with a crude mortality of 0.7 per 100 000 patients [9]. In the United States, gallbladder (GB) disease remains one of the most common inpatient diagnoses accounting for more than 260 000 hospital admissions and an annual health care provider expenditure exceeding $3.03 billion [10].

2.0. Pathogenesis of Acute Cholecystitis

Acute calculous cholecystitis (ACC) is an acute inflammation of the gallbladder, which in the majority of cases (90-95%) is precipitated by cystic duct obstruction caused by a gallstone [11].

Acute acalculous cholecystitis (AAC) occurs in the remaining 5-10% and develops in the absence of gallstones usually in the context of a severe illness. Many of these patients are thought to have cystic duct obstruction due to inspissated bile, cellular debris or local edema [12]. Other causes of cystic duct obstruction in AAC are cystic duct kinking, fibrosis, cystic duct compression by adhesive bands, anomalous vessels, lymphadenopathy and tumors [12]. Common conditions associated with AAC are presented in Table 1.

Table 1. Conditions associated with acute acalculous cholecystitis

Conditions
1. Ischemia
Coronary artery disease
Cardiopulmonary resuscitation
Heart failure
Shock
2. Bile stasis
Polytrauma
Recent surgery (cardiac, abdominal vascular, orthopaedic, etc)
Critical illness
Total parenteral nutrition
Dehydration
Mechanical ventilation
Prolonged opiate therapy
3. Bile composition change
Multiple blood transfusions
Resorption of large hematomas
4. Infection of the gallbladder
Bacterial
Mycobacterium tuberculosis (tuberculosis)
Salmonella enteritidis, typhi, Virchow (salmonellosis)
Coxiella burnetii (Q fever)
Brucella melitensis (brucellosis)
Leptospira interrogans (leptospirosis)
Vibrio cholerae (cholera)
Orientia tsutsugamushi (scrub typhus)
Fungal
Candidas albicans, torulopsis and glabrata (candidiasis)
Histoplasma capsulatum (histoplasmosis)

Table 1. (Continued)

Conditions
Viral
Cytomegalovirus
Hepatitis A
Epstein–Barr virus
5. Parasitic infestation
Cyclospora cayetanensis (cyclosporiasis)
Microsporidia (microsporidiosis)
Schistosoma mansonii (schistosomiasis)
Plasmodium falciparum and vivax (malaria)
6. Biliary obstruction (cystic duct, CBD)
Ampullary stenosis
Echinococcosis
Ascariasis
Primary and secondary tumors of gallbladder, cystic duct, CBD
7. Vasculitis
Systemic lupus erythemadosus
Polyarteritis nodosa
Chung-Strauss
Giant cell arteritis
Henoch-Schonlein purpura
8. Immunosuppression
Decreased CD4/CD8 ratio
Acute myelogenous leukemia
Immunosuppressive therapy
Acquired immunodeficiency syndrome
9. Miscellaneous
Diabetes mellitus
End-stage renal disease

The main trigger for AAC is thought to be the combination of direct ischemic injury to the gallbladder and bile stasis [13]. The gallbladder receives blood supply from the cystic artery which is a true terminal artery that has no anastomoses from other arteries. Therefore, any obstruction, interruption or reduction in blood supply to the gallbladder would render the gallbladder mucosa ischemic and trigger AAC.

Despite different triggers, ACC and AAC share a common pathogenesis that is the release of phospholipase A2 from the gallbladder epithelium with subsequent hydrolysis of bile lecithin to lysolecithin. Lysolecithin is a membrane-active cellular toxin that damages the protective glycoprotein layer of the mucosa and exposes epithelial cells to the detergent action of concentrated bile salts [14]. This leads to gallbladder dysmotility, gallbladder distention and an increase in intraluminal bile pressure. In turn, increased intraluminal bile pressure impairs blood supply to the gallbladder causing gallbladder wall ischemia, necrosis and perforation (Figure 1) [13, 14].

Initially, gallbladder inflammation is aseptic but subsequently, bacterial contamination develops and infective complications can include gallbladder empyema, suppurative cholecystitis, pericholecystic, hepatic abscesses and biliary sepsis.

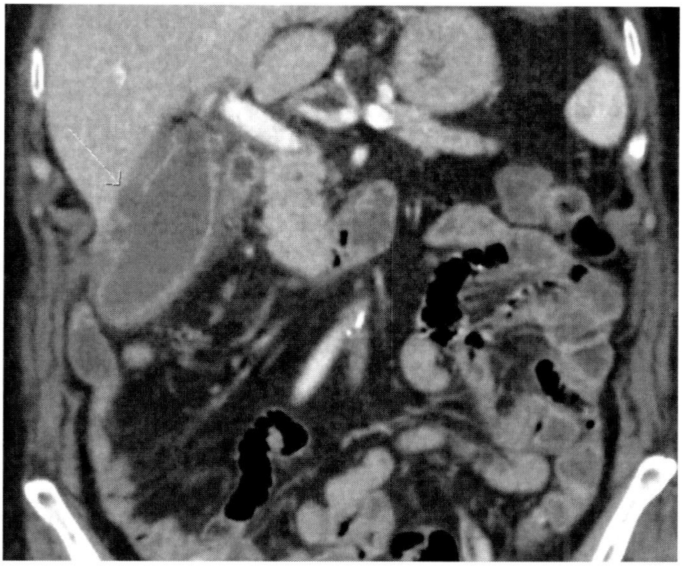

Figure 1. Coronal image from a computed tomographic scan of the abdomen shows gallbladder perforation (arrow).

3.0. Morphology of Acute Cholecystitis

3.1. Macroscopically

No specific morphological features distinguish between acute calculous and acute acalculous cholecystitis, except for the presence of gallstones. The gallstones may be contained within the lumen, but frequently, one becomes lodged in the gallbladder neck or cystic duct. Macroscopically, the gallbladder is often enlarged and tense. The serosal surface may show a variety of changes including congestion, hemorrhage and exudation, with discoloration ranging from bright red to deeply violaceous and black, depending on the extent of tissue necrosis and inflammation.

Inside the gallbladder findings may include bile sludge, turbid bile, blood, fibrin or frank pus. The presence of pus defines empyema of the gallbladder. The mucosa may be haemorrhagic and partially or completely sloughed. In cases of gangrenous cholecystitis, there is partial or complete necrosis of the gallbladder wall with or without accompanying perforation. Serosal exudate is often accompanied by adhesions between the gallbladder and adjacent bowel or omentum.

Exacerbations of AC may occur in patients with gallbladders which show histological evidence of previous ischemic insults or inflammation (acute on chronic cholecystitis). In these instances the gallbladder may be fibrosed and shrunken, or there may be fibrous adhesions to surrounding structures. Fibrous adhesions infer healed previous inflammatory episodes.

3.2. Microscopically

Histological differences characteristic of both ACC and AAC have been described, but there is significant overlap in these findings. Common histological findings include edema and hemorrhage in the gallbladder wall in early stages. There may be neutrophil margination in blood vessels. Ischemic injury to the mucosa is characterized by areas of mucosal ulceration or necrosis, followed by interstitial neutrophilic infiltration, accumulation of pus in the gallbladder wall and transmural necrosis. Within a few days of the onset of AC there is also a subserosal fibroblastic proliferation and abundant eosinophils may be seen during resolution of inflammation.

Acute exacerbations of chronic cholecystitis are characterized by neutrophilic mucosal infiltrates in a gallbladder which, also may have metaplastic mucosal changes, Aschoff-Rokitansky sinuses, transmural chronic inflammatory cells and serosal fibrosis (Figure 2).

Overall AC can be expected to go through the following four stages:

The First Stage, Days 2 to 4: Acute Edematous Cholecystitis (Figure 3)

In the earliest stages, the gallbladder wall, predominantly the subserosal layer, is edematous due to accumulation of interstitial fluid. Dilated and congested capillaries and lymphatics may be accompanied by areas of early interstitial hemorrhage.

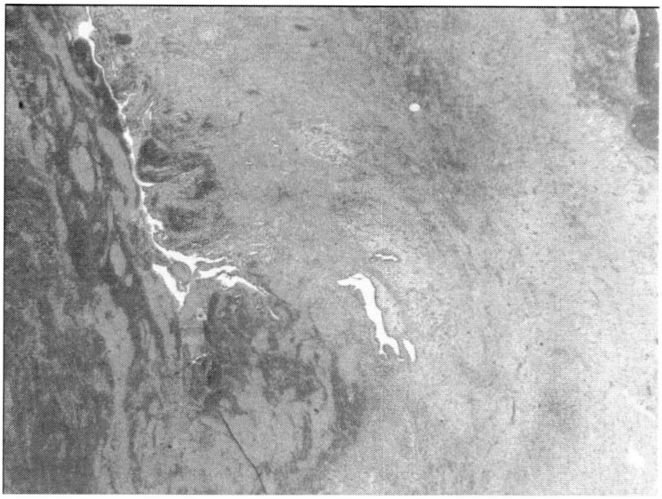

Figure 2. Low power view of a gallbladder with evidence of chronic cholecystitis (extensive fibrosis of the wall, transmural inflammation and epithelial sinuses) and superimposed acute cholecystitis (mucosal ulceration and hemorrhage).

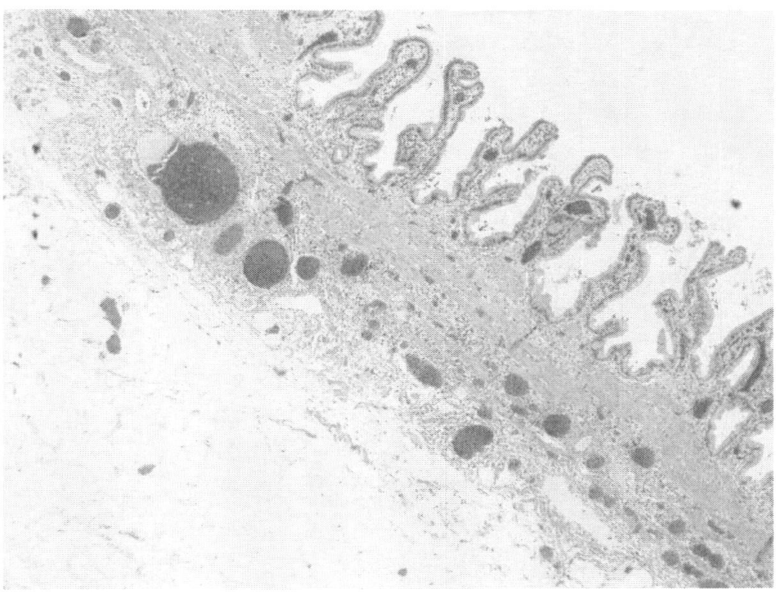

Figure 3. Histological changes in acute edematous cholecystitis.

The Second Stage, Days 3 to 5: Acute Necrotizing Cholecystitis (Figure 4)

In addition to vascular congestion and interstitial edema, neutrophils begin to infiltrate the surface epithelium and mucosal necrosis develops. The acute inflammatory response is mostly confined to the mucosa and does not involve the full thickness of the gallbladder wall.

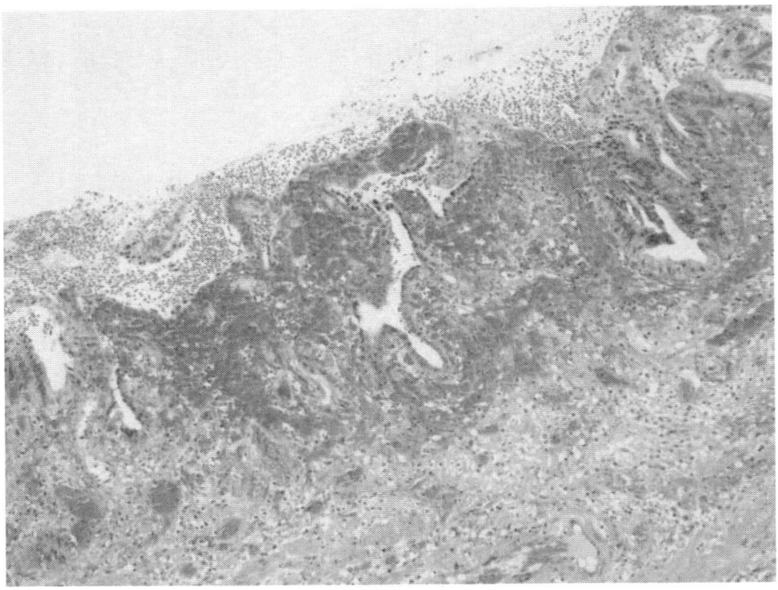

Figure 4. Histological changes in acute necrotizing cholecystitis.

The Third Stage, Days 7 to 10: Acute Suppurative Cholecystitis (Figure 5) and Acute Gangrenous Cholecystitis (Figure 6)

In the later stages of AC there is extension of areas of necrosis and inflammation to eventially involve the entire thickness of the gallbladder wall. If bacteria are present in the bile, then acute suppurative cholecystitis follows. The gallbladder may be distended with pus (empyema), or intramural and pericholecystic abscesses may form.

Gangrenous cholecystitis is a severe form of AC, which is more likely to occur in patients with co-morbidities such as old age, critical illness, cardiovascular disease, diabetes, etc. In this setting, gallbladder ischemia leads to coagulative tissue necrosis and decomposition. The gallbladder is characteristically distended with a hemorrhagic, violacous to black discoloured wall. Histologically, the mucosa and lamina muscularis are frequently absent and replaced by necrotic debris, neutrophils, and granulation tissue.

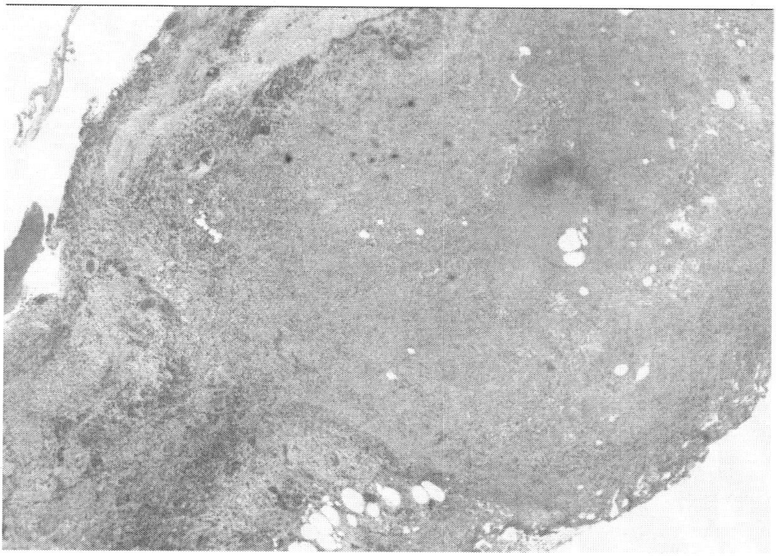

Figure 5. Histological changes in acute suppurative cholecystitis.

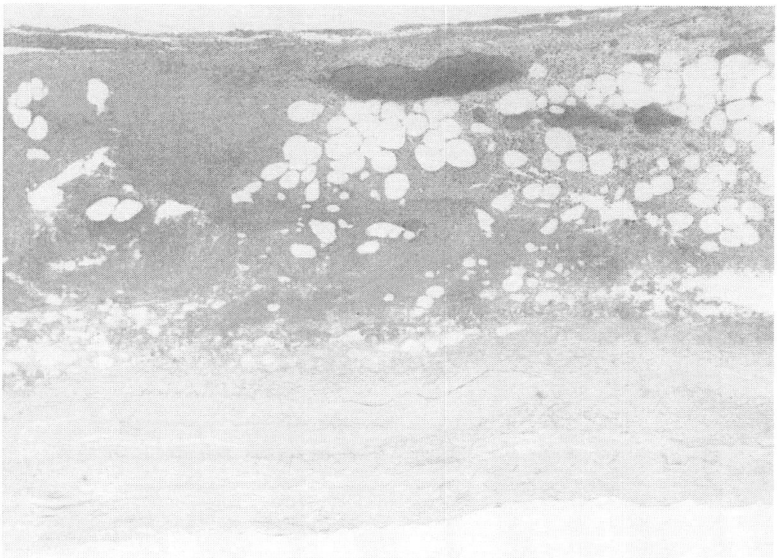

Figure 6. Histological changes in acute gangrenous cholecystitis.

On histological grounds alone, a clear distinction between severe/ extensive suppurative cholecystitis and gangrenous cholecystitis may not always be possible and may be subjective.

During the stage progression of acute cholecystitis the active repair process of inflammation becomes progressively more evident as thickening of the wall due to young scar tissue consisting of a tissue culture-like fibroblastic proliferation.

The Fourth Stage, beyond day 10: Pericholecystic Abscess (Figure 7) and Gallbladder Perforation (Figure 8).

Pericholecystic abscess is diagnosed when perforated suppurative cholecystitis is walled off by omental adhesions to contain the inflammatory process.

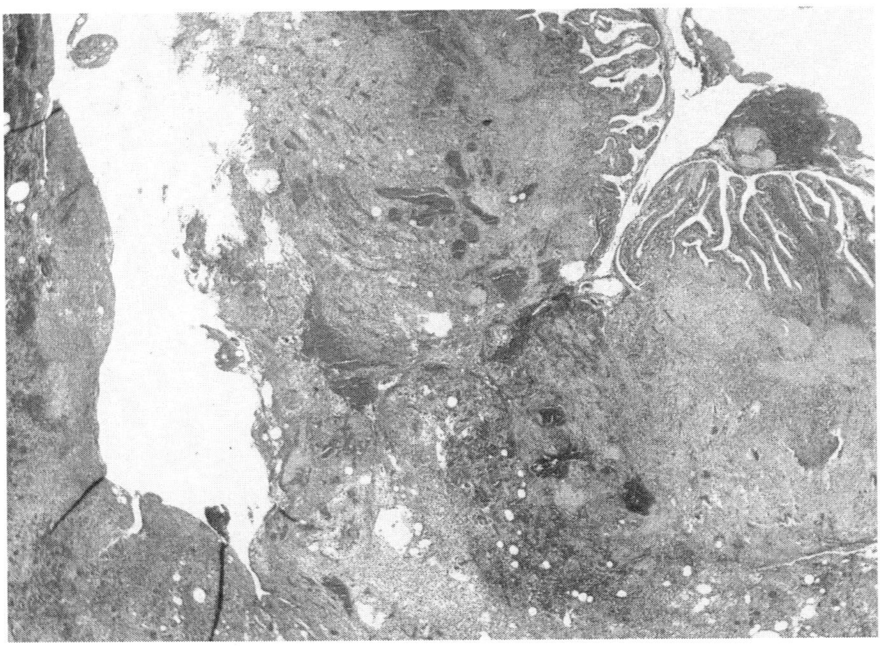

Figure 7. Peritoneal tissue or omentum is adherent to the gallbladder. In the angle between the tissue is a collection of inflammatory exudate with abundant neutrophils, consistent with a pericholecystic abscess.

Gallbladder perforation is characterized by transmural extension of suppurative or gangrenous cholecystitis with spill over of the exudate onto the serosal surface.

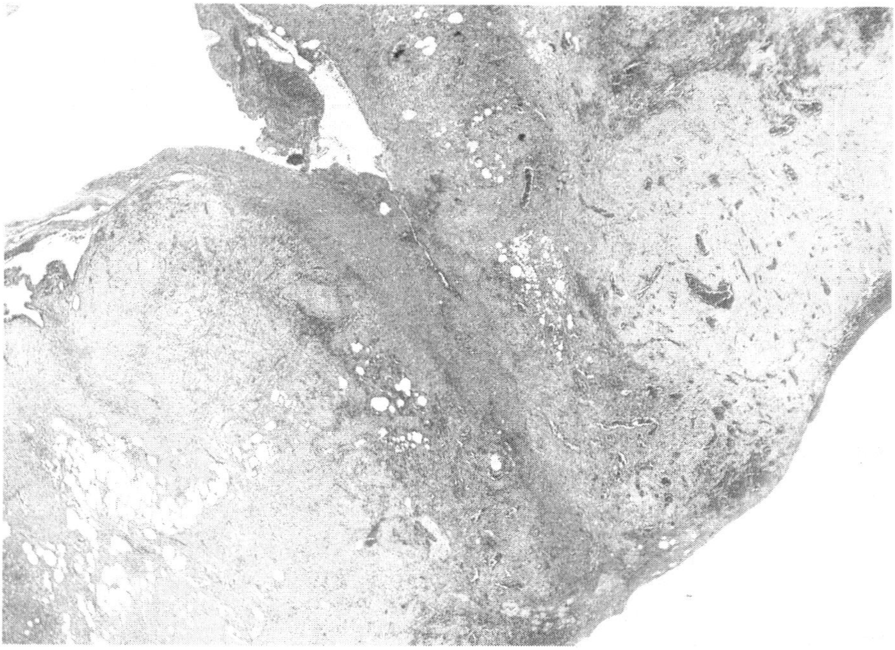

Figure 8. A tract of suppurative inflammation extends from the mucosal surface to the serosal surface, consistent with an area of perforation. In the background is active chronic cholecystitis.

4.0. Clinical Findings of Acute Cholecystitis

4.1. Symptoms and Clinical Signs

Patients with ACC commonly present with sudden onset of severe right upper quadrant (RUQ) or epigastric pain, nausea, vomiting, anorexia, diaphoresis and low-grade fever. High-grade fever, chills, rigors and signs of sepsis may also occur [15]. Abdominal pain is the most frequent symptom of AC and is present in about 80% of patients. RUQ/epigastric pain may radiate to the right scapula. Some patients report that RUQ pain increases with deep inspiration. An acute attack of abdominal pain is frequently precipitated by ingestion of a large or fatty meal. If untreated, pain may gradually subside over a period of 12-18 hours. Patients frequently report having had previous attacks of biliary colic.

Nausea and vomiting have been reported in 73% and 62% of patients with AC, respectively [16]. Fever is recorded in about 30% of patients with AC (body temperature > 37.5°C) [17].

Clinical symptoms of AAC tend to be more subtle and concealed by underlying conditions including severe trauma, recent surgery, sepsis or other critical illness that can precipitate the attack. A high index of suspicion is important for early diagnosis of AAC in critically ill patients, particularly those on ventilators, because, if left untreated, AAC is almost always associated with a fatal outcome [13].

Physical examination of patient reveals RUQ rebound tenderness in approximately 50% of patients, guarding in 30%, a palpable RUQ mass in 20% and positive Murphy's sign in 60% of patients with AC [16, 18]. Patients with perforated gallbladder and diffuse biliary peritonitis often have severe systemic signs that include fever, tachycardia, tachypnea, sweating and delirium. Physical examination elicits abdominal pain on coughing, percussion tenderness and guarding of the abdomen indicative of peritoneal irritation consistent with peritonitis.

4.2. Laboratory Findings

Elevated white cell count (WCC) has been demonstrated in 80% of patients with AC [15, 19]. In the remainder WCC is either normal or occasionally, patients may be leukopenic, especially in the presence of biliary sepsis (paper submitted for publication).

C-reactive protein (CRP) is known to be elevated in AC [20]. The level of CRP increases with progression of acute gallbladder inflammation from acute on chronic cholecystitis, acute edematous cholecystitis to pericholecystic abscess and AC with gallbladder perforation [20]. In a small subset of patients who present with AC soon after developing RUQ pain, the initial CRP can be normal [21]. Therefore, repeat testing 6-8 hours after presentation is helpful if clinical suspicion persists.

Liver function tests (serum bilirubin, alkaline phosphatase, gamma-glutamyl transferase, aspartate aminotransferase, alanine aminotransferase, albumin) and amylase are useful. Mild hyperbilirubinemia, mildly raised serum aminotransferases and amylase are common laboratory findings in AC. However, moderate elevation in serum total bilirubin and alkaline phosphatase concentration may indicate the presence of choledocholithiasis, Mirizzi syndrome or cholangitis and should prompt further investigation.

Serum electrolytes, urea, amylase and creatinine are important laboratory tests for grading the severity of AC, especially if the patient has fever, vomiting, diaphoresis and peritonism. Arterial blood gas analysis should be obtained in patients with hypotension, high-grade fevers, acute pancreatitis and generalised peritonitis.

Coagulation studies (partial thromboplastin time, prothrombin time) are frequently performed particularly if interventions are planned such as surgery, percutaneous drainage or endoscopic retrograde cholangiography (ERC).

4.3.0. Imaging Studies

The 2007 Tokyo criteria were modified in 2013 to reflect the importance of imaging in the diagnosis of acute cholecystitis. Ultrasound (US) is the initial imaging modality of choice because of expediency, wide availability in most hospitals, lack of radiation exposure and ease of performance at the bedside [22, 23]. Accuracy can be limited by factors such as ultrasonographer skills and patient cooperation, but US remains the preferred imaging modality in patients with suspected acute cholecystitis.

4.3.1. Ultrasound

The classic US appearance of gallstones is echogenic foci with posterior acoustic shadowing [24]. Their visibility is usually enhanced by hypoechoic surrounding bile. Important sonographic findings in the diagnosis of AC include tenderness when pressure is applied over the gallbladder to elicit a positive sonographic Murphy sign, marked distention of the gallbladder (gallbladder long axis diameter more than 80 mm, short axis diameter above 40 mm), gallbladder wall thickening of more than 4 mm, a sonolucent halo in the gallbladder wall, and pericholecystic fluid (Figure 7) [24-27].

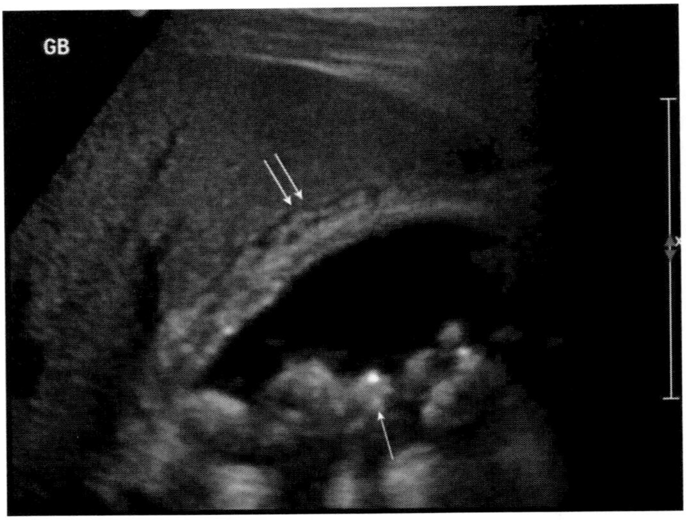

Figure 9. US appearance in a patient with acute calculous cholecystitis demonstrates dependent gallstones (single arrow) in a thick walled gallbladder with a sonolucent rim (double arrow). The gallbladder was tender to probe pressure.

Reported sensitivities for US have varied. In 2011, Van Randen reported a sensitivity of 73% (95% CI: 61% - 85%) in diagnosing AC with a specificity of 97% (95% CI: 96% - 98%), a positive predictive value of 37% (95% CI: 22% - 51%) and a negative predictive value of 96% (95% CI: 95% - 97%) [28]. An emergency department physician-performed US study reported sensitivity up to 96% and specificity of 79% [29]. The use of US is limited in uncooperative patients, patients with a large body habitus or gaseous abdominal distention and is not sensitive in identifying common bile duct (CBD) stones [30]. Ultrasound technology continues to evolve and accuracy in diagnosis is clearly improved when US is combined with other clinical and laboratory markers of inflammation [31]. In challenging cases, US is frequently supplemented with CT scanning, magnetic resonance imaging (MRI) or cholescintigraphy [30]. However, these techniques are secondary problem solving modalities in the investigation of patients with suspected AC.

4.3.2. Computed Tomography

Multi-detector computed tomography (CT) is more likely to be used as the initial imaging modality in patients presenting with abdominal pain that is not typical for AC, in those with more generalized abdominal pain and, in many departments, after hours when CT is more readily available than US [32-34].

In ACC, important CT findings include gallbladder wall thickening, pericholecystic stranding, gallbladder distention, gallbladder subserosal edema, and pericholecystic fluid (Figure 10) [35]. In acute acalculous cholecystitis the most frequent CT findings are gallbladder wall thickening and enlargement of the gallbladder [35]. Other less common CT findings include high-attenuation bile and gallbladder subserosal edema [35].

In diagnosing AC, CT has a reported sensitivity of 73% (95% CI: 61% - 85%), a specificity of 98% (95% CI: 97% - 99%, a positive predictive value of 51% (95% CI: 36% - 67%) and a negative predictive value of 96% (95% CI: 95% - 98%), values which are similar to those that have been reported for US [28]. CT is particularly valuable in obese patients and for patients with complications of AC, including gangrenous, emphysematous and hemorrhagic cholecystitis, gallbladder perforation and gallstone ileus [36]. CT is well known to be less sensitive than both US and MRI for identifying gallstones, particularly bilirubin stones which can be isodense with bile. CT is also known to underestimate gallbladder wall thickening [33, 34]. The accuracy of unenhanced helical CT in detecting CBD stones is less than US with a reported sensitivity of 65% (95% confidence interval (CI): 44% - 82%), a specificity of 84% (95% CI: 63% - 95%), positive predictive value of 81% (95% CI: 57% - 94%), and a negative predicted value of 70% (95% CI: 50% - 85%) [37]. However, it is important to recognize these features of AC on unenhanced CT scans which are likely to be performed when renal colic is suspected clinically and in patients with renal impairment. CT can be performed rapidly with reduced scanning time compared with MRI which contributes to greater patient acceptance. The main concern with using CT, particularly in younger patients is the radiation exposure. A CT scan increases the effective radiation exposure, on average, by 21.5 mSv per patient [38]. A 2-year cumulative radiation exposure greater than 100 mSv with a life expectancy exceeding 15 years increases the risk of radiation-induced leukemia and solid-tumor cancers by more than 3% [39].

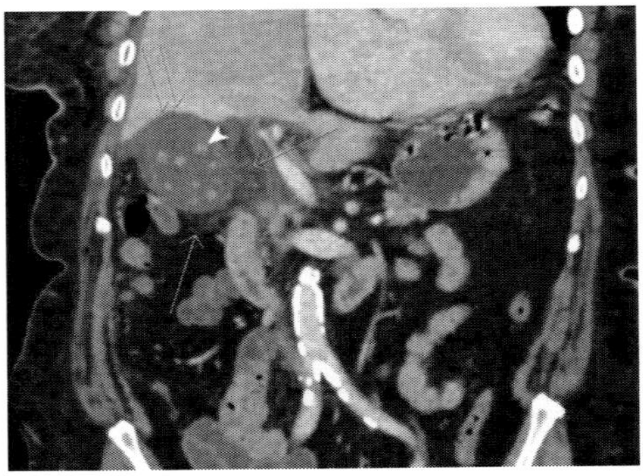

a

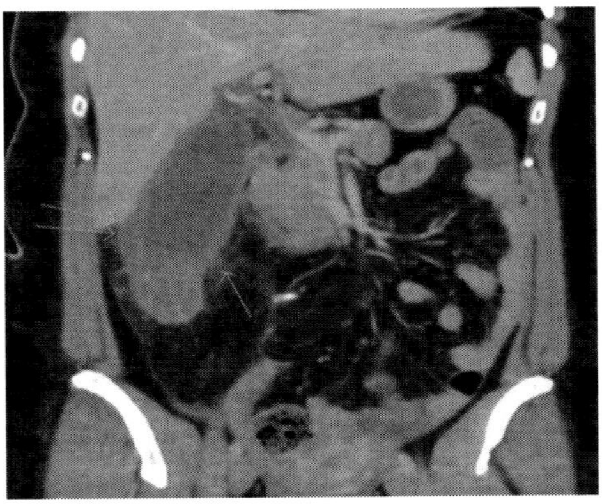

b

Figure 10A (coronal plane), figure 10B (sagittal plane). CT appearance of acute calculous cholecystitis shows multiple gallstones (arrowhead), a distended gallbladder with a thickened wall (double arrow) and adjacent stranding in the surrounding fat (single arrow).

4.3.3. Magnetic Resonance Imaging

Magnetic resonance imaging (MRI) is the safest secondary imaging modality for pregnant patients with abdominal pain after US. MR cholangiopancreatography is also particularly useful for patients with obstructive jaundice due to CBD stones, which can be missed on both US due to overlying bowel gas and on CT which depends on increased Hounsfield units for stone detection. MR cholangiography depicts the dilated biliary tract without the need for gadolinium and is the most accurate imaging modality for diagnosing biliary stones with reported sensitivity of 96% (95% CI: 78% -

99%), specificity of 100% (95% CI: 84% - 100%), positive predictive value of 100% (95% CI: 83-100%), and negative predictive value of 96% (95% CI 78% - 100%) [37]. Predictably, MR cholangiography is significantly more sensitive for CBD stones than CT ($p = 0.008$), but has a similar specificity [37].

MRI findings of uncomplicated AC include gallbladder distension, stones in the cystic duct or gallbladder neck, intraluminal sludge, gallbladder wall thickening, increased enhancement of the gallbladder wall, pericholecystic fluid, abnormal signal intensity and edematous stratification in the gallbladder wall (Figure 9) [33]. T2-weighted HASTE (half-Fourier acquisition single shot turbo-spin echo) MRI using pericholecystic high signal intensity has an accuracy of 89% of diagnosing AC, a sensitivity of 91%, a specificity of 79%, a positive predicted value of 87% and a negative predicted value of 85% [40]. MRI has been used in the diagnosis of complicated forms of AC, including acute gangrenous cholecystitis, gallbladder perforation and pericholecystic abscess [33].

Compared with CT, MRI is more sensitive in the diagnosis of AC using findings of gallbladder wall thickening, gallstones and gallbladder wall hyperemia. MRI is also better able to depict gallbladder wall vascular deficiency, and effectively shows adjacent liver hyperemia ($p = 0.004 - 0.063$) [41]. In addition, MRI has been reported to be more effective than CT in demonstrating pericholecystic inflammatory fat stranding ($p = 0.016$) [41]. Although these findings suggest a better overall performance of MRI than abdominal CT in identifying AC, MRI is rarely available in the emergency department setting. Furthermore, the extra time required for MR scanning, patient compliance (particularly those who may be claustrophobic) and limited access of medical teams to patients who may be systemically unwell are all factors which limit the role of MRI in the acute setting of AC.

MRI is contraindicated in patients with epicardial and temporary transvenous pacing leads, pulmonary artery hemodynamic monitoring/ thermodilution catheters (such as Swan-Ganz catheters), intra-aortic balloon pumps, ventricular-assist devices [42, 43]. Permanent cardiac pacemakers and implantable cardioverter-defibrillators are strong relative contraindications to MRI [42]. Despite the risk of gadolinium induced nephropathy being rare, MRI contrast agents are discouraged in patients with severe renal impairment (estimated glomerular filtration rate<30ml/min per 1.73 m^2) [44]. Severe claustraphobia which may require sedation can preclude this imaging modality in up to 15% of patients [43].

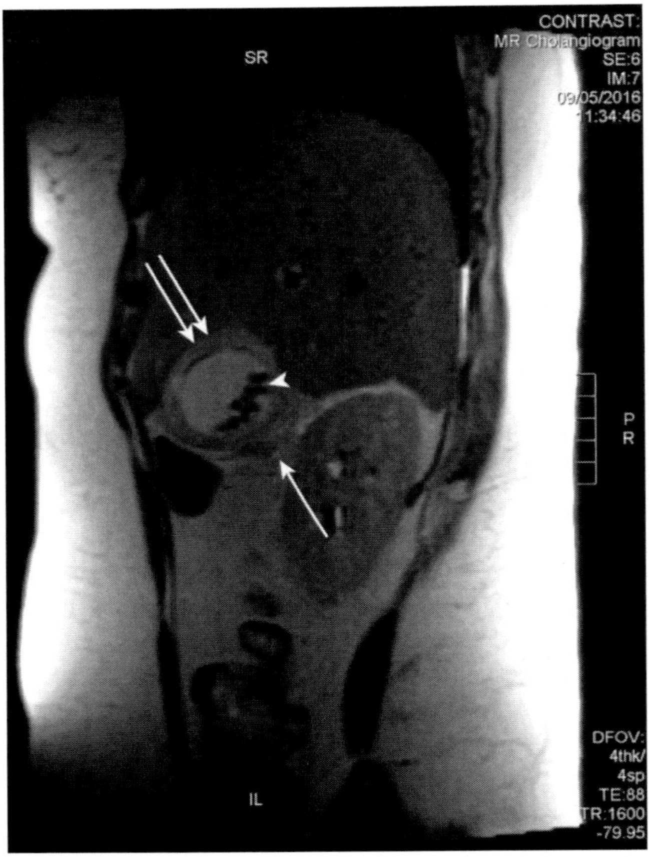

Figure 11. Coronal MRI image shows gallstones (arrowhead) within a thick walled gallbladder (double arrow) and adjacent stranding (single arrow).

4.3.4. Cholescintigraphy

Cholescintigrapy using 99mTc-hepatic iminodiacetic acid (HIDA) has been reported in the past as an accurate diagnostic modality in AC. 99mTc-HIDA injected intravenously is absorbed by hepatocytes and excreted into bile. Cholecystitis can be demonstrated either by nonvisualization of the gallbladder or by poor gallbladder contractility. Absence of imaging of the gallbladder within 60 mins is indicative of cystic duct obstruction and AC [45]. Non-visualization of the gallbladder for AC has a sensitivity of 94%, specificity of 17%, a positive predictive value of 83%, a negative predictive value of 40%, a likelihood ratio for positive results of 113% and a likelihood ratio for negative results of 35% [46].

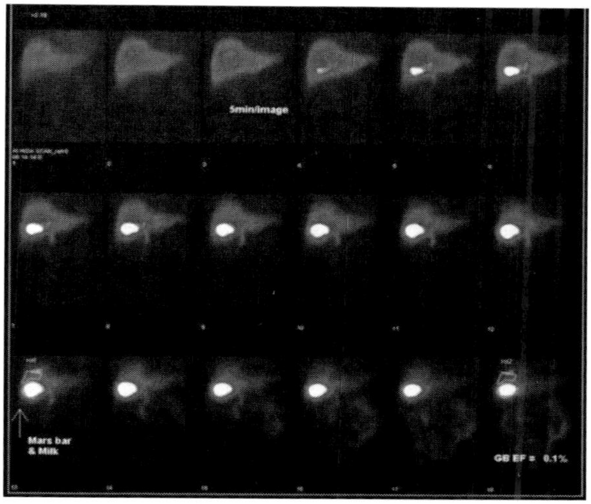

a

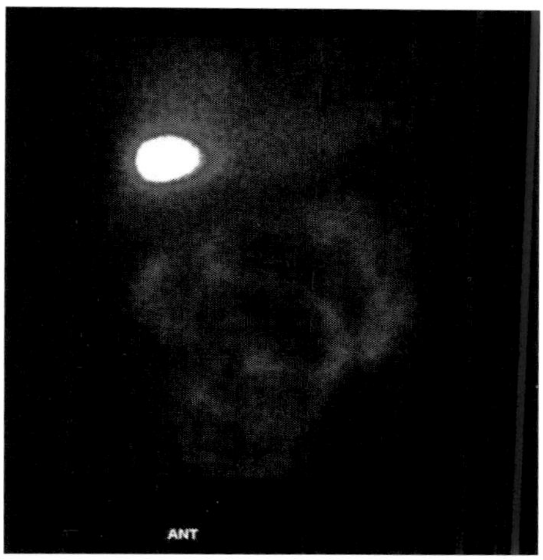

b

Figure 12A, B. HIDA scan after a fat stimulus given at 60 min to a patient with acute acalculous cholecystitis shows poor contractility of the gallbladder with Tc 99 remaining within the lumen after 90 min.

In HIDA scans, patients with patent cystic ducts may result in a false-negative finding for AC [12]. AAC patients with patent cystic ducts will have reduced gallbladder ejection fraction stimulated by sincalide or a fatty meal, but this will not differentiate them from patients with chronic cholecystitis (Figure 12) [12]. If the rim sign is present, it will confirm the diagnosis of AC.

Otherwise, radiolabeled leukocytes, 99mTc-hexamethylpropyleneamine oxime leucocytes, can be helpful [48].

Another cholescintigraphy finding in AC is the "rim sign" that is a rim of increased pericholecystic hepatic activity. Bushnell at al. showed that the cholescintigraphic rim sign was statistically associated with the histological diagnosis of AC [47]. In AC the rim sign has 61% sensitivity and 95% specificity. When the rim sign is combined with non-visualized gallbladder at one hour, the positive predicted value for AC is 94% [47].

Reported sensitivities for cholescintigraphy 96% (95% CI: 94% to 97%) in the diagnosis of AC are significantly higher than those for both US (81%; 95% CI: 75% - 87%) ($p < 0.001$) and MRI (85%; 95% CI: 66% - 95%) ($p = 0.03$) [48]. Specificity of cholescintigraphy (90%; 95% CI: 86% - 93%) is similar to those of US (83%; 95% CI: 74% - 89%) ($p = 0.06$) and MRI (81%; 95% CI: 69% - 90%) ($p = 0.07$) [48]. Significant constraints of cholescintigraphy are limited availability especially after hours, longer examination time of up to four hours and significantly higher costs. Therefore, scintigraphy is largely superceded by US, CT and MRI in the diagnosis of acute cholecystitis but remains useful for identifying gallbladder contractility dysfunction, particularly in the absence of gallstones.

5.0. Misdiagnosis of Acute Cholecystitis without Use of CRP as a Diagnostic Criterion

Despite advances in imaging, preoperative diagnosis of AC, especially acute gangrenous cholecystitis (AGC), remains challenging and may result in misdiagnosis [49-51]. In a nonfasted patient, the gallbladder can be collapsed and the wall appears thickened on imaging. Brook et al. reported 14 cases of AC misdiagnosed on both US and CT scans [50]. In their study, US findings resulted in 3 (21%) overcalls, when chronic cholecystitis, hepatitis and urinary sepsis were diagnosed as AC. These misdiagnoses resulted in one unnecessary percutaneous cholecystostomy and in another, cholecystectomy. There were 5 (36%) undercalls that resulted in delayed management, development of AGC, gallbladder perforation and death [50]. In 6 patients (43%), CT was reported to undercall patients with AC and this lead to gallbladder perforation, acute renal failure and an increased risk of peri-operative complications, including intra-abdominal hemorrhage and bile leakage [50].

Late diagnosis and treatment of AC leads to development of more severe grades of AC, formation of extensive adhesions around the gallbladder and marked inflammatory reaction in Calot's triangle. These pathological changes make laparoscopic cholecystectomy (LC) technically a more challenging procedure and predispose patients to an increased likelihood of conversion to open surgery (CTO), subtotal cholecystectomy that in some patients might require re-operation, and an increased risk of perioperative complications [52-54]. AC untreated for longer than 72 hours is associated with a threefold increase in the risk of CTO (OR 3.1; 95% CI: 1.2 – 7.7; p = 0.0072) [55].

To prevent complications due to misdiagnosis, Kiviluoto et al. proposed an early operative approach to all symptomatic patients due to gallstones [56]. However, it is unrealistic to expect that all patients with symptomatic gallbladder stone disease will undergo cholecystectomy during their index hospital admission due to significant health care constraints. Lack of prioritization for emergency, acute and delayed elective surgery would defer surgery in many other patients with advanced forms of AC and predisposes them to an increased risk of peri-operative complications, which include deterioration in their general medical conditions, CTO and intra-abdominal organ injury such as bile duct injury during LC. This potentially increases patients' length of the index hospital admission. Failure to perform cholecystectomy for AC in elderly patients is associated an increased mortality [57]. Compared with patients who underwent cholecystectomy for AC during their index hospital admission, those who did not have surgery had a higher 2-year surgery or gallstone-related hospital readmission, 4.4 and 38%, respectively (p < 0.0001) [57]. Hospital readmission for gallstone-related complications is associated with an increased rate of open cholecystectomy and an additional US $7000 Medicare payment per admission [57].

6.0. The 2007 and 2013 Tokyo Guidelines for Acute Cholecystitis

To improve the accuracy of diagnosing AC, members of the 2006 Tokyo International Consensus Meeting defined the diagnostic criteria for AC, known as the 2007 Tokyo Guidelines (TG07), and included elevated C-reactive protein (CRP) as a diagnostic benchmark of AC [58].

CRP is an acute-phase protein produced by hepatocytes in response to an increased secretion of interleukin-6 (IL-6) by macrophages in infection, inflammation, trauma, necrosis and malignancy [59]. IL-6 triggers the transcription factors C/EBP family members, STAT3 and NF-κB that attach to the CRP gene, located on the short arm of chromosome 1, and induces its transcription and synthesis of a CRP molecule [60]. CRP is a potent opsonin that binds with a high affinity to phosphocholine residues and other autologous and extrinsic ligands expressed on surfaces of damaged host cells and bacterial microorganisms, and recruits the complement initiator C1q which activates the classical complement pathway [61]. Surfaces of injured host and microbial cells become opsonized with C3b and C5b complement components. C1q and C3b on the surface of bacteria, necrotic and apoptotic cells are recognized by specific receptors on macrophages. This receptor-ligant interaction enhances phagocytosis and intracellular killing of target cells by macrophages [62, 63]. C5b together with C6, C7, C8, and C9 assembles in a lipophilic multi-molecular unit, the membrane-attack complex, with formation of a transmembrane lytic channel and a subsequent extracellular lysis of target cells [62]. CRP is a very sensitive systemic marker of tissue injury and inflammation. Concentration of CRP starts rising in 6 hours after onset of a pathological condition [59, 64]. The plasma half-life of CRP is about 19 hours and largely determined by the rate of CRP hepatic synthesis [61].

Table 2. Proposed modifications to the 2013 Tokyo guidelines diagnostic criteria for acute cholecystitis (modified from [16])

A. Local signs of inflammation etc.:
(1) Murphy's sign, (2) RUQ mass/pain/tenderness
B. Systemic signs of inflammation etc.:
(1) Fever, (2) raised WBC, (3) leucopenia (WBC < 4000/mm³), (4) elevated CRP
C. Imaging findings: imaging findings characteristic of acute cholecystitis
Suspected diagnosis: At least one item in A + at least one item in B
Definite diagnosis: At least one item in A + at least one item in B + C

Acute hepatitis and other acute abdominal diseases should be excluded

Abbreviations: RUQ, right upper quadrant, CRP, C-reactive protein, WBC, white blood count

In 2013 TG07 for AC were revised. In TG13 for AC, a greater emphasis is placed upon diagnostic imaging characteristic of AC (Table 2) [58]. To further improve the accuracy of diagnosing AC, we proposed using leucopenia (WCC < 4000/mm^3) as an additional analytic bench mark. Modified TG13 diagnostic criteria for AC are presented in Table 2.

Table 3. Cutoff values and areas under receiver operating characteristic curve of WCC and CRP in acute cholecystitis (modified from [20])

Histopathology of acute cholecystitis	WCC cutoff (95% CI) x 10^9/L	CRP cutoff (95% CI), mg/L	AUC of WCC (95% CI)	AUC of CRP (95% CI)	P-value
All forms of AC	9.15 (8.7-9.6)	30.5 (10.2-50.8)	0.83 (0.79-0.87)	0.94 (0.92-0.97)	<0.00005
TG13 mild AC	9.0 (8.6-9.4)	26.5 (12.7-40.3)	0.76 (0.70-0.82)	0.9 (0.86-0.94)	<0.0001
TG13 moderate-severe AC¥	11.1 (9.7-12.4)	57.5 (43.7-71.3)	0.9 (0.85-0.94)	0.98 (0.96-1.0)	0.0003
Acute on chronic cholecystitis	9.15 (8.81 - 9.49)	26.5 (15.72 - 37.28)	0.72 (0.65 - 0.79)	0.87 (0.82 - 0.92)	0.0004
Acute edematous cholecystitis	9.05 (8.29 - 9.81)	30.5 (3.34 - 51.68)	0.78 (0.69 - 0.87)	0.93 (0.87 - 0.99)	0.0001
Acute necrotizing cholecystitis	9.05 (6.97 - 11.12)	57.5 (34.74 - 80.26)	0.89 (0.83 - 0.95)	0.97 (0.94 - 1.0)	0.0149
Acute suppurative cholecystitis	9.15 (7.96 - 10.34)	92 (76.43 - 111.57)	0.82 (0.67 - 0.97)	1.0 (1.0 - 1.0)	0.0189
Acute gangrenous cholecystitis	11.65 (10.63 - 12.67)	67 (61.78 - 72.22)	0.93 (0.89 - 0.98)	0.99 (0.97 - 1.0)	0.0375
Pericholecystic abscess/gallbladder perforation with biliary peritonitis	9.15 (7.82 - 10.48)	86 (66.28 - 105.72)	0.89 (0.76 - 1.0)	1.0 (1.0 - 1.0)	0.0852

¥ includes acute necrotizing, suppurative, gangrenous cholecystitis, gallbladder torsion, pericholecystic abscess, gallbladder perforation with biliary peritonitis

In a retrospective multi-center study TG13 diagnostic criteria for AC had 94% accuracy, 91.2% sensitivity, 96.9% specificity, 96.7% positive predicted value, 91.6% negative predictive value, 29.2% positive likelihood ratio and 0.1% negative likelihood ratio [65]. However, CRP is not yet used routinely for the diagnosis of AC in the USA, Canada, Europe and other countries [21, 49, 66-70].

Recently, the diagnostic significance of CRP in AC has been demonstrated [20]. We showed that CRP has a better discriminative power than WCC in the histological diagnosis of acute on chronic cholecystitis, acute edematous, necrotizing, suppurative and gangrenous cholecystitis (Table 3).

CRP and WCC performed equally well in pericholecystic abscess and gallbladder perforation with biliary peritonitis [20]. In all histological forms of AC combined, the cutoff value of WCC in diagnosing AC was 9.15 (95% CI: 8.7 – 9.6) x 10^9/L. Sensitivity at the cutoff point of WCC was 73%, specificity 76%, and the area under receiver operating characteristic curve (AUC) of WCC at the cutpoint was 74%.

The CRP cutoff concentration in diagnosing AC was 30.5 (95% CI: 10.2 – 50.8) mg/L. The sensitivity of CRP at the cutoff point was 85%, specificity 92%, and the AUC at the cutoff point 89%. Comparison of the AUC of WCC (AUC = 83%, 95% CI: 0.79 – 0.87) and the AUC of CRP (AUC = 94%, 95% CI: 0.92 – 0.97) demonstrated a better discriminative power of CRP (chi2(1) = 27.29, $p < 0.00005$) (Figure 11).

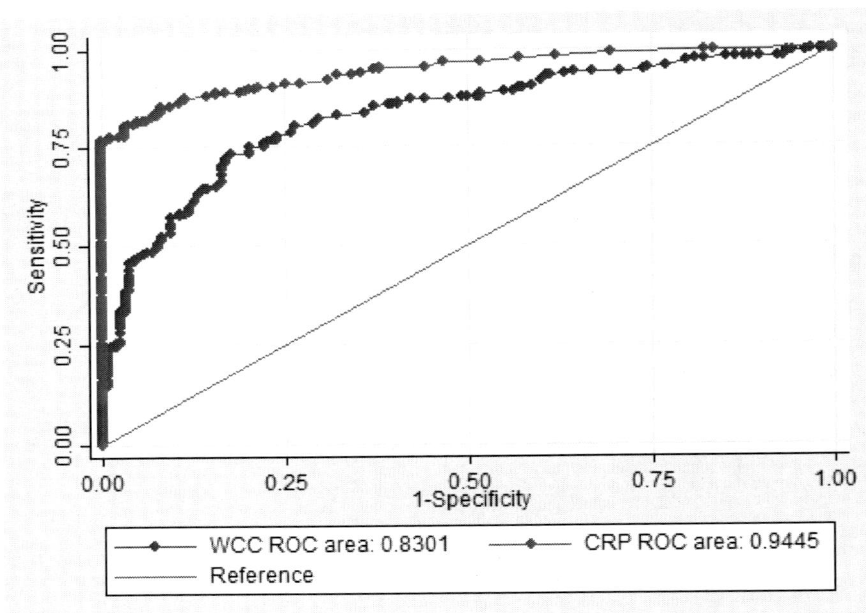

Figure 13. ROC curves of WCC and CRP in the overall diagnosis of acute cholecystitis.

7.0. SEVERITY GRADES OF ACUTE CHOLECYSTITIS

To refine surgical and antimicrobial management of AC the TG07 and TG13 for AC divides AC into severity grades: mild (grade I) AC, moderate (grade II) AC and severe (grade III) AC (Table 4) [16, 58].

Table 4. The 2013 Tokyo guidelines severity grading for acute cholecystitis (adapted from [16])

Grade I (mild) acute cholecystitis
Does not meet the criteria of "Grade III" or "Grade II" acute cholecystitis. Grade I can also be defined as acute cholecystitis in a healthy patient with no organ dysfunction and mild inflammatory changes in the gallbladder, making cholecystectomy a safe and low-risk operative procedure.
Moderate (grade II) acute cholecystitis
Grade II (moderate) acute cholecystitis
Associated with any one of the following conditions:
1. Elevated white blood count (>18000/mm^3)
2. Palpable tender mass in the right upper quadrant
3. Duration of complaints > 72 h
4. Marked local inflammation (gangrenous cholecystitis, pericholecystic abscess, hepatic abscess, biliary peritonitis, emphysematous cholecystitis)
Grade III (severe) acute cholecystitis
Associated with dysfunction of any one of the following organs/systems:
1. Cardiovascular dysfunction (hypotension requiring treatment with dopamine ≥5mcg/kg/min, or any dose of norepinephrine)
2. Neurological dysfunction (decreased level of consciousness)
3. Respiratory dysfunction (PaO2/FiO2 ratio < 300)
4. Renal dysfunction (oliguria, creatinine > 2.0 mg/dL)
5. Hepatic dysfunction (PT-INR> 1.5)
6. Hematological dysfunction (platelet count < 100 000/mm^3)

The TG07/TG13 defining criterion for mild (grade I) AC is effortlessness and safety of LC, whereas the moderate-severe (grades II-III) AC among other diagnostic criteria is characterised by difficult dissection. When the operating surgeon encounters a difficult laparoscopic dissection, CTO is advised to prevent intra-abdominal organ injury, including bowel and bile duct injury. Emergency CTO is used to control intra-abdominal hemorrhage and to repair iatrogenic injuries that incurred during LC [55].

TG13 severity grading criteria for mild and moderate-severe AC are arbitrary and incomplete. The TG13 diagnostic criterion for moderate AC, elevated WCC (>18000/m³) is lacking a discriminative power for CTO [71]. AC patients with WCC > 18000/m³ have the same risk for CTO as those with WCC ≤ 18000/m³ (OR = 1.1; 95% CI: 0.3 - 3.3; p = 0.511) [55].

Discriminative power of moderate AC criterion "Palpable tender mass in the right upper quadrant" is still unknown.

The TG13 diagnostic criterion "Duration of complaints > 72 hours" has been demonstrated to predict CTO. In Asai's study, 12 (41.4%) of 29 patients in the CTO group and 36 (18.4%) of 196 patients in the LC group had duration of complaints for longer than 72 hours (p = 0.0004) [71]. Therefore, patients with duration of complaints more than 72 hours have a three-fold increased risk of CTO (OR 3.1; 95% CI: 1.2 – 7.7; p = 0.0072) [55].

The TG13 criterion of moderate AC Marked local inflammation (biliary peritonitis, pericholecystic abscess, hepatic abscess, gangrenous cholecystitis, emphysematous cholecystitis) is vague, imprecise and open to interpretation. It is not clear whether these criteria refer to clinical, radiological or histological findings.

Another limitation of the TG13 for AC severity grading is the absence of CRP as a diagnostic criterion in mild, moderate and severe categories. As a result, surgeons continue providing the same treatment to all AC patients on the basis of their history, physical examination findings, clinical and laboratory response to antibacterial therapy, intravenous fluids and analgesics. Recently, it has been shown that CRP measurement is not associated with improved management of AC patients [21]. Compared with the group of AC patients without CRP measurement, patients from the CRP measurement group had a higher proportion of acute gangrenous cholecystitis, 18/145 (12.4%) patients against 63/269 (23.4%) patients, respectively, p = 0.007, but a longer time to operation theatre, median time 45.8 hours (range: 1.8-270.3 hours) and 52.9 hours (range: 0.9-370.1 hours), respectively, p = 0.024 [21].

Recently, we have shown that there is an association between histological severity of AC and CTO (Table 5).

Therefore, according to the TG07/TG13 defining criterion for mild and moderate-severe AC that is effortlessness and safety of LC, acute on chronic cholecystitis and acute edematous cholecystitis have a low rate of CTO and comprise the mild AC group, whereas acute necrotizing, suppurative, gangrenous cholecystitis, pericholecystic abscess and AC with gallbladder perforation constitute the moderate-severe AC group. Compared with the mild AC group, patients with moderate-severe AC had a two-fold increase in rate of CTO (Relative risk = 1.6; 95% CI: 1.1-2.2; p = 0.008) (paper submitted for publication).

Table 5. Conversion of laparoscopic cholecystectomy to open surgery in different histological diagnoses of acute cholecystitis

Gallbladder histopathology	CTO rate, (%)	RR	95% CI	P-value*
Acute on chronic cholecystitis	38/202 (18.8)	1	---	---
Acute edematous cholecystitis	13/69 (18.8)	1	0.57-1.77	0.996
Acute necrotizing cholecystitis	26/70 (37.1)	1.97	1.3-3.0	0.001
Acute suppurative cholecystitis	1/6 (16.7)	0.9	0.14-5.42	0.896
Acute gangrenous cholecystitis¥	29/84 (34.5)	1.84	1.22-2.77	0.004
Pericholecystic abscess/ acute cholecystitis with gallbladder perforation	1/3 (33.3)	2.4	1.08-5.18	0.032

¥ includes one case of gallbladder torsion

Abbreviations: CTO, laparoscopic cholecystectomy converted to open surgery; RR, relative risk; CI, confidence interval.

7.1. Diagnostic Levels of WCC and CRP in Mild and Moderate-Severe AC

7.1.2. Mild (Grade I) AC

The optimal cutoff value of WCC in diagnosing mild AC was 9.0 (95% CI: 8.6 – 9.4). Sensitivity at the cutoff point was 64%, specificity 75%, and the AUC at the cutpoint was 70% (Table 2). CRP cutoff value in diagnosing mild AC was 26.5 (95% CI: 12.7 – 40.3). Sensitivity at the cutoff point was 76%, specificity 88%, and the AUC at the cutoff point 82%.

7.1.3. Moderate-Severe (Grade II-III) AC

The optimal cutoff value of WCC in diagnosing moderate-severe AC was 11.1 (95% CI: 9.7 – 12.4) x 10^9/L (Table 2). Sensitivity at the cutpoint was 75%, specificity 91%, and AUC at the cut-off point 83%. The optimal cutoff of CRP was 57.5 (95% CI: 43.7 – 71.3) mg/L. Sensitivity at the cutoff point was 94%, specificity 100%, the AUC at the cutoff point 97%.

7.2. Use of Inflammatory Biomarkers in Predicting Severity of AC

We evaluated the association between biomarkers of inflammation; leucopenia (WCC<4000/mm^3), leucocytosis (WCC>11000/mm^3) and elevated

CRP, and severity of AC (mild, moderate-severe). We found that the combination of two abnormal biomarkers (abnormal WCC and raised CRP) was associated with more advanced forms of AC whereas in patients with normal WCC and normal levels of CRP (0 number of positive biomarkers) the histologic grades of AC were least severe (ch2(2) = 19.6; p <0.0005). Those patients with only one elevated biomarker, (either leucopenia, leucocytosis, or raised CRP) were more likely to be in the mild category than the moderate-severe category of AC (Table 6).

Table 6. An association between abnormal WCC and raised CRP and severity of AC

Inflammatory biomarkers	Mild AC, N=119, n (%)	Moderate-severe AC, N=59, n (%)
0	6 (5)	0 (0)
1	59 (49.6)	12 (20.3)
2	54 (45.4)	47 (79.7)

0 biomarker means normal WCC and CRP; 1 biomarker signifies the presence of either leucopenia, leucocytosis, or raised CRP; 2 biomarkers denote the presence of abnormal WCC and elevated CRP.

CONCLUSION

The definitive diagnosis of ACC is based on clinical history, physical examination findings, laboratory investigations and imaging studies. CRP has better discriminative powers than WCC and is a useful marker both in diagnosing AC and as an indicator of severity. Concentration of CRP exceeding 44 mg/L indicates a grade of moderate-severe AC. The presence of more than one inflammatory biomarkers is also associated with more severe grades of AC. We propose that combinations of systemic signs of inflammation should be used not only as diagnostic criteria but also to indicate the severity of AC. This warrants further evaluation in prospective studies.

Mild and moderate-severe grades of AC can be determined not only on the basis of gallbladder histology but also on their biomarkers and clinical behaviour. These grades are associated with different risks of CTO. Acute on chronic and acute edematous cholecystitis constitute mild AC based on low rate of CTO. Moderate-severe AC consists of patients with histological evidence of acute necrotizing, suppurative and gangrenous cholecystitis as well as those who develop complications such as pericholecystic abscess and gallbladder perforation.

REFERENCES

[1] Glambek I, Kvaale G, Arnesjo B, Soreide O. Prevalence of gallstones in a Norwegian population. *Scand J Gastroenterol.* [Research Support, Non-U.S. Gov't]. 1987 Nov;22(9):1089-94.

[2] Muhrbeck O, Ahlberg J. Prevalence of gallstone disease in a Swedish population. *Scand J Gastroenterol.* [Research Support, Non-U.S. Gov't]. 1995 Nov;30(11):1125-8.

[3] Everhart JE, Khare M, Hill M, Maurer KR. Prevalence and ethnic differences in gallbladder disease in the United States. *Gastroenterology.* 1999 Sep;117(3):632-9.

[4] Gracie WA, Ransohoff DF. The natural history of silent gallstones: the innocent gallstone is not a myth. *N Engl J Med.* 1982 Sep 23;307(13):798-800.

[5] Halldestam I, Enell EL, Kullman E, Borch K. Development of symptoms and complications in individuals with asymptomatic gallstones. *Br J Surg.* 2004 Jun;91(6):734-8.

[6] Friedman GD. Natural history of asymptomatic and symptomatic gallstones. *Am J Surg.* [Research Support, U.S. Gov't, P.H.S. Review]. 1993 Apr;165(4):399-404.

[7] Papadakis M, Ambe PC, Zirngibl H. Critically ill patients with acute cholecystitis are at increased risk for extensive gallbladder inflammation. *World J Emerg Surg.* 2015;10:59.

[8] Haltmeier T, Benjamin E, Inaba K, Lam L, Demetriades D. Early versus delayed same-admission laparoscopic cholecystectomy for acute cholecystitis in elderly patients with comorbidities. *J Trauma Acute Care Surg.* 2015 Apr;78(4):801-7.

[9] Peery AF, Dellon ES, Lund J, Crockett SD, McGowan CE, Bulsiewicz WJ, et al. Burden of gastrointestinal disease in the United States: 2012 update. *Gastroenterology.* [Research Support, N.I.H., Extramural Research Support, Non-U.S. Gov't]. 2012 Nov;143(5):1179-87 e1-3.

[10] Russo MW, Wei JT, Thiny MT, Gangarosa LM, Brown A, Ringel Y, et al. Digestive and liver diseases statistics, 2004. *Gastroenterology.* [Research Support, Non-U.S. Gov't Research Support, U.S. Gov't, P.H.S.]. 2004 May;126(5):1448-53.

[11] Kimura Y, Takada T, Strasberg SM, Pitt HA, Gouma DJ, Garden OJ, et al. TG13 current terminology, etiology, and epidemiology of acute cholangitis and cholecystitis. *J Hepatobiliary Pancreat Sci.* [Review]. 2013 Jan;20(1):8-23.

[12] Ziessman HA. Hepatobiliary scintigraphy in 2014. *J Nucl Med.* [Review]. 2014 Jun;55(6):967-75.

[13] Crawford JM. The liver and biliary tract. In: Cotran RS, Kumar, V., Collins, T., editor. Robbins pathologic basis of disease. Sixth ed. Philadelphia: W.B. Saunders Company; 1999. p. 845-929.

[14] Suriawinata AA, Thung SN. The liver and biliary system. In: Strayer DS, Rubin, E.,, editor. Rubin's pathology: clinicopathologic foundations of medicine. Seventh ed. Philadelphia: *Wolters Kluwer Health;* 2015. p. 825-85.

[15] Smith EA, Dillman JR, Elsayes KM, Menias CO, Bude RO. Cross-sectional imaging of acute and chronic gallbladder inflammatory disease. *AJR Am J Roentgenol.* [Review]. 2009 Jan;192(1):188-96.

[16] Yokoe M, Takada T, Strasberg SM, Solomkin JS, Mayumi T, Gomi H, et al. TG13 diagnostic criteria and severity grading of acute cholecystitis (with videos). *J Hepatobiliary Pancreat Sci.* [Practice Guideline]. 2013 Jan;20(1):35-46.

[17] Schofield PF, Hulton NR, Baildam AD. Is it acute cholecystitis? *Ann R Coll Surg Engl.* 1986 Jan;68(1):14-6.

[18] Eskelinen M, Ikonen J, Lipponen P. Contributions of history-taking, physical examination, and computer assistance to diagnosis of acute small-bowel obstruction. A prospective study of 1333 patients with acute abdominal pain. *Scand J Gastroenterol.* [Clinical Trial Controlled Clinical Trial Multicenter Study]. 1994 Aug;29(8):715-21.

[19] Alponat A, Kum CK, Koh BC, Rajnakova A, Goh PM. Predictive factors for conversion of laparoscopic cholecystectomy. *World J Surg.* 1997 Jul-Aug;21(6):629-33.

[20] Beliaev AM, Marshall RJ, Booth M. C-reactive protein has a better discriminative power than white cell count in the diagnosis of acute cholecystitis. *J Surg Res.* 2015 Sep;198(1):66-72.

[21] Beliaev AM, Booth M. C-reactive protein measurement is not associated with an improved management of acute cholecystitis: a plie for a change. *J Surg Res.* 2015 Sep;198(1):93-8.

[22] Yarmish GM, Smith MP, Rosen MP, Baker ME, Blake MA, Cash BD, et al. ACR appropriateness criteria right upper quadrant pain. *J Am Coll Radiol.* 2014 Mar;11(3):316-22.

[23] Zenobii MF, Accogli E, Domanico A, Arienti V. Update on bedside ultrasound (US) diagnosis of acute cholecystitis (AC). *Intern Emerg Med.* 2015 Nov 4.

[24] Carroll BA. Preferred imaging techniques for the diagnosis of cholecystitis and cholelithiasis. *Ann Surg.* [Review]. 1989 Jul;210(1):1-12.

[25] Bree RL. Further observations on the usefulness of the sonographic Murphy sign in the evaluation of suspected acute cholecystitis. *J Clin Ultrasound.* 1995 Mar-Apr;23(3):169-72.

[26] Ralls PW, Halls J, Lapin SA, Quinn MF, Morris UL, Boswell W. Prospective evaluation of the sonographic Murphy sign in suspected acute cholecystitis. *J Clin Ultrasound.* 1982 Mar;10(3):113-5.

[27] Martinez A, Bona X, Velasco M, Martin J. Diagnostic accuracy of ultrasound in acute cholecystitis. *Gastrointest Radiol.* 1986;11(4):334-8.

[28] van Randen A, Lameris W, van Es HW, van Heesewijk HP, van Ramshorst B, Ten Hove W, et al. A comparison of the accuracy of ultrasound and computed tomography in common diagnoses causing acute abdominal pain. *Eur Radiol.* [Comparative Study Research Support, Non-U.S. Gov't]. 2011 Jul;21(7):1535-45.

[29] Torres-Macho J, Anton-Santos JM, Garcia-Gutierrez I, de Castro-Garcia M, Gamez-Diez S, de la Torre PG, et al. Initial accuracy of bedside ultrasound performed by emergency physicians for multiple indications after a short training period. *Am J Emerg Med.* [Clinical Trial]. 2012 Nov;30(9):1943-9.

[30] Williams EJ, Green J, Beckingham I, Parks R, Martin D, Lombard M. Guidelines on the management of common bile duct stones (CBDS). *Gut.* [Practice Guideline Review]. 2008 Jul;57(7):1004-21.

[31] Juvonen T, Kiviniemi H, Niemela O, Kairaluoma MI. Diagnostic accuracy of ultrasonography and C reactive protein concentration in acute cholecystitis: a prospective clinical study. *Eur J Surg.* 1992 Jun-Jul;158(6-7):365-9.

[32] Harvey RT, Miller WT, Jr. Acute biliary disease: initial CT and follow-up US versus initial US and follow-up CT. *Radiology.* [Comparative Study]. 1999 Dec;213(3):831-6.

[33] Tonolini M, Ravelli A, Villa C, Bianco R. Urgent MRI with MR cholangiopancreatography (MRCP) of acute cholecystitis and related complications: diagnostic role and spectrum of imaging findings. *Emerg Radiol.* [Review]. 2012 Aug;19(4):341-8.

[34] Shakespear JS, Shaaban AM, Rezvani M. CT findings of acute cholecystitis and its complications. AJR *Am J Roentgenol.* [Review]. 2010 Jun;194(6):1523-9.

[35] Fidler J, Paulson EK, Layfield L. CT evaluation of acute cholecystitis: findings and usefulness in diagnosis. *AJR Am J Roentgenol.* 1996 May;166(5):1085-8.

[36] Pinto F, Pinto A, Russo A, Coppolino F, Bracale R, Fonio P, et al. Accuracy of ultrasonography in the diagnosis of acute appendicitis in adult patients: review of the literature. *Crit Ultrasound J.* 2013 Jul 15;5 Suppl 1:S2.

[37] Soto JA, Alvarez O, Munera F, Velez SM, Valencia J, Ramirez N. Diagnosing bile duct stones: comparison of unenhanced helical CT, oral contrast-enhanced CT cholangiography, and MR cholangiography. *AJR Am J Roentgenol.* [Comparative Study]. 2000 Oct;175(4):1127-34.

[38] Jones AC, Woldemikael D, Fisher T, Hobbs GR, Prud'homme BJ, Bal GK. Repeated computed tomographic scans in transferred trauma patients: Indications, costs, and radiation exposure. *J Trauma Acute Care Surg.* [Research Support, Non-U.S. Gov't]. 2012 Dec;73(6):1564-9.

[39] Zoli S, Trabattoni P, Dainese L, Annoni A, Saccu C, Fumagalli M, et al. Cumulative radiation exposure during thoracic endovascular aneurysm repair and subsequent follow-up. *Eur J Cardiothorac Surg.* 2012 Aug;42(2):254-59; discussion 9-60.

[40] Regan F, Schaefer DC, Smith DP, Petronis JD, Bohlman ME, Magnuson TH. The diagnostic utility of HASTE MRI in the evaluation of acute cholecystitis. Half-Fourier acquisition single-shot turbo SE. *J Comput Assist Tomogr.* [Clinical Trial Comparative Study Randomized Controlled Trial]. 1998 Jul-Aug;22(4):638-42.

[41] Kaura SH, Haghighi M, Matza BW, Hajdu CH, Rosenkrantz AB. Comparison of CT and MRI findings in the differentiation of acute from chronic cholecystitis. *Clin Imaging.* [Case Reports Comparative Study Evaluation Studies]. 2013 Jul-Aug; 37(4):687-91.

[42] Levine GN, Gomes AS, Arai AE, Bluemke DA, Flamm SD, Kanal E, et al. Safety of magnetic resonance imaging in patients with cardiovascular devices: an American Heart Association scientific statement from the Committee on Diagnostic and Interventional Cardiac Catheterization, Council on Clinical Cardiology, and the Council on Cardiovascular Radiology and Intervention: endorsed by the American College of Cardiology Foundation, the North American Society for Cardiac

Imaging, and the Society for Cardiovascular Magnetic Resonance. *Circulation.* 2007 Dec 11;116(24):2878-91.

[43] Dill T. Contraindications to magnetic resonance imaging: non-invasive imaging. *Heart.* [Review]. 2008 Jul;94(7):943-8.

[44] Bongartz G. Imaging in the time of NFD/NSF: do we have to change our routines concerning renal insufficiency? *Magma.* [Editorial Review]. 2007 Apr;20(2):57-62.

[45] Katabathina VS, Zafar AM, Suri R. Clinical Presentation, Imaging, and Management of Acute Cholecystitis. *Tech Vasc Interv Radiol.* 2015 Dec;18(4):256-65.

[46] Bohdiewicz PJ. The diagnostic value of grading hyperperfusion and the rim sign in cholescintigraphy. *Clin Nucl Med.* 1993 Oct;18(10):867-71.

[47] Bushnell DL, Perlman SB, Wilson MA, Polcyn RE. The rim sign: association with acute cholecystitis. *J Nucl Med.* 1986 Mar;27(3):353-6

[48] Kiewiet JJ, Leeuwenburgh MM, Bipat S, Bossuyt PM, Stoker J, Boermeester MA. A systematic review and meta-analysis of diagnostic performance of imaging in acute cholecystitis. *Radiology.* [Meta-Analysis Review]. 2012 Sep;264(3):708-20.

[49] Wu B, Buddensick TJ, Ferdosi H, Narducci DM, Sautter A, Setiawan L, et al. Predicting gangrenous cholecystitis. *HPB* (Oxford). 2014 Mar 17.

[50] Brook OR, Kane RA, Tyagi G, Siewert B, Kruskal JB. Lessons learned from quality assurance: errors in the diagnosis of acute cholecystitis on ultrasound and CT. *AJR: Am J Roentgenol.* 2011 March;196(3):597 - 604.

[51] Yacoub WN, Petrosyan M, Sehgal I, Ma Y, Chandrasoma P, Mason RJ. Prediction of patients with acute cholecystitis requiring emergent cholecystectomy: a simple score. *Gastroenterol Res Pract.* 2010;2010:901739.

[52] Elshaer M, Gravante G, Thomas K, Sorge R, Al-Hamali S, Ebdewi H. Subtotal cholecystectomy for "difficult gallbladders": systematic review and meta-analysis. *JAMA Surg.* [Meta-Analysis Review]. 2015 Feb;150(2):159-68.

[53] Strasberg SM, Pucci MJ, Brunt LM, Deziel DJ. Subtotal Cholecystectomy-"Fenestrating" vs "Reconstituting" Subtypes and the Prevention of Bile Duct Injury: Definition of the Optimal Procedure in Difficult Operative Conditions. *Journal of the American College of Surgeons.* 2016 Jan;222(1):89-96.

[54] Jayant M, Kaushik R. Presentation and management of gallbladder remnant after partial cholecystectomy. *Trop Gastroenterol.* 2013 Apr-Jun;34(2):99-103.

[55] Beliaev AM, Booth M. Risk factors and predictive models for conversion of laparoscopic cholecystectomyt to open surgery, and surgical quality outcome measures. In: Garbuzenko D, editor. *Emergency Abdominal Surgery.* Rijeka: InTech; 2016.

[56] Kiviluoto T, Siren J, Luukkonen P, Kivilaakso E. Randomised trial of laparoscopic versus open cholecystectomy for acute and gangrenous cholecystitis. *Lancet.* [Clinical Trial Comparative Study Randomized Controlled Trial]. 1998 Jan 31;351(9099):321-5.

[57] Riall TS, Zhang D, Townsend CM, Kuo Y-F, Goodwin J, S,. Failure to perform cholecystectomy for acute cholecystitis in elderly patients is associated with increased morbidity, mortality and costs. *J Am Coll Surg.* 2010 May;210(5):668 - 79.

[58] Hirota M, Takada T, Kawarada Y, Nimura Y, Miura F, Hirata K, et al. Diagnostic criteria and severity assessment of acute cholecystitis: Tokyo Guidelines. *J Hepatobiliary Pancreat Surg.* [Practice Guideline Research Support, Non-U.S. Gov't]. 2007;14(1):78-82.

[59] Pepys MB, Hirschfield GM. C-reactive protein: a critical update. *J Clin Invest.* [Research Support, Non-U.S. Gov't Review]. 2003 Jun;111(12):1805-12.

[60] Black S, Kushner I, Samols D. C-reactive Protein. *J Biol Chem.* [Review]. 2004 Nov 19;279(47):48487-90.

[61] Vigushin DM, Pepys MB, Hawkins PN. Metabolic and scintigraphic studies of radioiodinated human C-reactive protein in health and disease. *J Clin Invest.* [Research Support, Non-U.S. Gov't]. 1993 Apr;91 (4):1351-7.

[62] Walport MJ. Complement. First of two parts. *N Engl J Med.* [Review]. 2001 Apr 5;344(14):1058-66.

[63] Walport MJ. Complement. Second of two parts. *N Engl J Med.* [Research Support, Non-U.S. Gov't Review]. 2001 Apr 12;344 (15):1140-4.

[64] Mihlan M, Blom AM, Kupreishvili K, Lauer N, Stelzner K, Bergstrom F, et al. Monomeric C-reactive protein modulates classic complement activation on necrotic cells. *Faseb J.* [Research Support, Non-U.S. Gov't]. 2011 Dec;25(12):4198-210.

[65] Yokoe M, Takada T, Strasberg SM, Solomkin JS, Mayumi T, Gomi H, et al. New diagnostic criteria and severity assessment of acute

cholecystitis in revised Tokyo Guidelines. *J Hepatobiliary Pancreat Sci.* [Practice Guideline]. 2012 Sep;19(5):578-85.

[66] Strasberg SM. Clinical practice. Acute calculous cholecystitis. *N Engl J Med.* [Review]. 2008 Jun 26;358(26):2804-11.

[67] Gutt CN, Encke J, Koninger J, Harnoss JC, Weigand K, Kipfmuller K, et al. Acute cholecystitis: early versus delayed cholecystectomy, a multicenter randomized trial (ACDC study, NCT00447304). *Ann Surg.* [Comparative Study Multicenter Study Randomized Controlled Trial Research Support, Non-U.S. Gov't]. 2013 Sep;258(3):385-93.

[68] Hwang H, Marsh I, Doyle J. Does ultrasonography accurately diagnose acute cholecystitis? Improving diagnostic accuracy based on a review at a regional hospital. *J Can Chir. juin* 2014;57(3):162-68.

[69] Nikfarjam M, Shen L, Fink MA, Muralidharan V, Starkey G, Jones RM, et al. Percutaneous cholecystostomy for treatment of acute cholecystitis in the era of early laparoscopic cholecystectomy. *Surg Laparosc Endosc Percutan Tech.* 2013 Oct;23(5):474-80.

[70] Furtado R, Page PL, Dunn G, Falk GL. High rate of common bile duct stones and postoperative abscess following percutaneous cholecystostomy. *Ann R Coll Surg Engl.* 2016 Jan 7:1-5.

[71] Asai K, Watanabe M, Kusachi S, Matsukiyo H, Saito T, Kodama H, et al. Risk factors for conversion of laparoscopic cholecystectomy to open surgery associated with the severity characteristics according to the Tokyo guidelines. *Surg Today.* 2014 Jan 29.

Biographical Sketch

Name: Andrei M. Beliaev

Affiliation: Green Lane Cardiothoracic Surgical Unit, Auckland City Hospital, Auckland, New Zealand

Education: Altay State Medical University, Barnaul city, Russia (1979-1985). M.D. at the Research Institute of Circulation Pathology, Novosibirsk, Russia (1991)

Address: Cardiothoracic Surgical Unit, Auckland City Hospital, Private Bag 92024, Auckland, New Zealand

Email AndreiB@adhb.govt.nz

Research and Professional Experience: Completed and Ongoing Research Projects and Clinical Audits: 1. Antihypoxic organism protection in open heart surgery under deep hypothermic cardiac arrest by intracranial hemostasia prevention and blood loss compensation, 2. Cost-effectiveness of allogeneic red blood cell transfusion, 3. Mortality risk factors in severely anemic Jehovah's Witness patients, 4. Refining screening criteria for blunt cerebro-vascular injury, 5. Cholecystectomies clinical audit at North Shore Hospital, Auckland, New Zealand. 6. Effect of socio-economic status in indigenous New Zealand population on lung transplant outcome and survival (ongoing).

Professional Appointments: Registrar

Honors: Royal Australasian College of Surgeons. Winner 2013 Best paper by a Trainee in Trauma Surgery at Royal Australasian College of Surgeons, ASC 2013 Auckland.

Publications Last 3 Years:

1. Beliaev AM, Shapkov P, Booth M. Incidence of gallbladder torsion in acute cholecystectomy patients. *ANZ J Surg*. 2015 Oct;85(10):793.
2. Beliaev AM, Booth M. C-reactive protein measurement is not associated with an improved management of acute cholecystitis: a plié for a change. *J Surg Res*. 2015 Sep;198(1):93-8.
3. Beliaev AM, Fougere C Thoracic outlet syndrome secondary to a mid-clavicle malunion. *BMJ Case Rep*. 2015 Jun 4;2015. pii: bcr2015209583. doi: 10.1136/bcr-2015-209583.
4. Beliaev AM, Marshall RJ, Booth M.C-reactive protein has a better discriminative power than white cell count in the diagnosis of acute cholecystitis. *J Surg Res*. 2015 Sep;198(1):66-72.
5. Beliaev AM, Booth M Prevalence of duplicate gallbladder in cholecystectomy patients. *ANZ J Surg*. 2015 Jan;85(1-2):96-7.
6. Beliaev AM, Booth M.Late two-stage laparoscopic cholecystectomy is associated with an increased risk of major bile duct injury. *ANZ J Surg*. 2016 Jan;86(1-2):63-8.
7. Beliaev AM, Beaven T, Koya MP Spontaneous passage of a very large ureteral stone. *ANZ J Surg*. 2014 Aug 12. doi: 10.1111/ans.12805. [Epub ahead of print].

8. Beliaev AM, Civil I. Multidetector CT angiography influences the choice of treatment for blunt carotid artery injury. *BMJ Case Rep.* 2014 Aug 6;2014. pii: bcr2013200659. doi: 10.1136/bcr-2013-200659.
9. Bisleri U, Beliaev AM. CT coronary angiography evaluation of involvement of the left internal mammary artery graft in advanced left upper lobe lung tumour. *BMJ Case Rep.* 2014 Mar 4;2014. pii: bcr2013202060. doi: 10.1136/bcr-2013-202060.
10. Beliaev AM, Roberts SA, Pemberton J, Haydock DA. Propionibacterium acnes biofilm endocarditis requiring radical cardiac debridement and prosthetic valve replacements. *ANZ J Surg.* 2015 Oct;85(10):787-8.
11. Beliaev AM, Barber PA, Marshall RJ, Civil I. Denver screening protocol for blunt cerebrovascular injury reduces the use of multi-detector computed tomography angiography. *ANZ J Surg.* 2014 Jun;84(6):429-32.
12. Beliaev AM, Civil I. Asymptomatic carotid blunt cerebrovascular injury: a new screening criterion. *ANZ J Surg.* 2014 Jun;84(6):491-2.
13. Karpenko AA, Ignatenko PV, Beliaev AM. Hybrid in situ replacement for Samson group V Staphylococcus aureus aortic graft infection. *BMJ Case Rep.* 2013 Jul 29;2013. pii: bcr2013010289. doi: 10.1136/bcr-2013-010289.
14. Beliaev AM, Mundy I. Bilateral simultaneous testicular torsion presenting as a diagnostic dilemma. *BMJ Case Rep.* 2013 May 22;2013. pii: bcr2013010137. doi: 10.1136/bcr-2013-010137.
15. Beliaev AM. High-risk anaemic Jehovah's Witness patients should be managed in the intensive care unit. *Blood Transfus.* 2013 Jul;11 (3):330-2.
16. Beliaev AM, Marshall RJ, Smith W, Windsor JA. Treatment monitoring and mortality risk adjustment in anaemic Jehovah's Witnesses. *ANZ J Surg.* 2013 Mar;83(3):161-4.
17. Beliaev AM, Allen SA. Chapter 4: Management and outcomes in severe anemia. In: Handbook of nutrition and diet in leukemia and blood disease therapy. Human Health Handbook no 12. R. R. Watson and D. Mahadevan (eds). - DOI 10.3920/978-90-8686-822-3_4. Wageningen Academic Publishers 2016

18. Beliaev AM, Booth M. C-reactive protein as a diagnostic and prognostic marker of acute cholecystitis. In: *Advances in Medicine and Biology. Nova Science Publishers,* 2016 (in press).

19. Beliaev AM, Booth M. Risk factors and predictive models for conversion of laparoscopic cholecystectomy to open surgery, and surgical quality outcome measures. In: *Emergency Abdominal Surgery.* Rijeka, Croatia, 2016 (in press).

20. Beliaev AM, Booth M. An association between conversion of laparoscopic cholecystectomy to open surgery and intra-abdominal organ injury. *ANZ J. Surg*. 2016; doi: 10.1111/ans.13539.

In: Acute Cholecystitis
Editor: Lisa Powell

ISBN: 978-1-63485-744-4

Chapter 4

TREATMENT FOR ACUTE CHOLECYSTITIS: EARLY AND DELAYED CHOLECYSTECTOMY

Miguel Sánchez-Carrasco[1], MD, PhD, Francisco Javier Sánchez-Manuel[1], MD, PhD, Adel Eldabe[1], MD, Fernando Martín-Acebes[1], MD, PhD, Federico Castillo-Suescun[2], MD, PhD and Juan Carlos Rodríguez-Sanjuán[2], MD, PhD

[1]Department of Surgery, Burgos University Hospital, Burgos, Spain
[2]Department of Surgery,
University Hospital "Marqués de Valdecilla," Santander, Spain

ABSTRACT

Acute cholecystitis is a pathological entity of inflammatory origin, with a high prevalence worldwide. Therefore, an appropriate diagnostic and therapeutic approach has important medical and socio-economic impact. There are two different alternatives for the surgical management of acute cholecystitis: early cholecystectomy during the index admission, within 72 hours from the onset of symptoms if possible, or delayed cholecystectomy during a later scheduled admission 4-6 weeks after a successful conservative treatment. Early cholecystectomy reduces days of hospital stay, hospital readmissions and seems to lead to a reduction in direct hospital costs. Only 50% of patients from delayed cholecystectomy will get their elective operation after the index episode, leaving half of the cases at risk of complications and mortality. Laparoscopic approach seems to be as safe as open surgery. Subtotal cholecystectomy may have the advantage of avoiding bile duct injury, and could decrease conversions rate in laparoscopic procedures.

Keywords: acute cholecystitis, early cholecystectomy, delayed cholecystectomy

ABBREVIATIONS

EC: Early cholecystectomy
DC: Delayed cholecystectomy
AC: Acute cholecystitis.

INTRODUCTION

AC is a pathological entity of inflammatory origin, usually associated with gallstones. It poses a significant socioeconomic problem in our society. In general, the definitive treatment is cholecystectomy, and there are two different options: EC during the index admission or DC during a later scheduled admission.

EPIDEMIOLOGY

The prevalence of asymptomatic gallstones in the western world is around 9% in men and 15% in women, reaching up to 25% over the age of 50 (Bateson MC, 1984). Most people who harbor gallstones are asymptomatic. Nearly 20% of asymptomatic cases will turn symptomatic during the following 15 years. Once initial symptoms appear, the risk of developing recurrent attacks is roughly 30% per year for the first two years, and the risk of complications is about 3% per year (Nahrwold DL, 1976. Bateson MC, 1984. Thistle JL, 1984. Friedman GD, 1989. Ransohoff DF, 1993. Kallo AN, 2001). Complications of gallstones include AC, stone migration to the bile ducts, with or without cholangitis, and gallstone pancreatitis, the most frequent being AC, carrying a risk of 6% to 11% over a median follow-up of 7 to 11 years (Friedman GD, 1993). Once complications arise, the odds of developing additional, and often more severe, complications are about 30% per year (Nahrwold DL, 1976. Bateson MC, 1984. Thistle JL, 1984. Friedman GD, 1989. Ransohoff DF, 1993. Kallo AN, 2001).

Pathophysiology

Aside from calculous AC, other forms of AC include: (1) acalculous, (2) xanthogranulomatous, (3) emphysematous, and (4) torsion of the gall bladder (Kimura Y, 2007).

It has been demonstrated that the mere obstruction of the cystic duct by stone or sludge is not enough to unleash the events leading to acute inflammation on its own (Morris CR, 1952. Roslyn JJ, 1980); the presence of a mucosal irritating agent is also necessary (Roslyn JJ, 1980). Contrary to what might be expected, bile culture studies are positive in only 22 to 46% of patients with biliary disease. The most common isolated species are Escherichia coli, Enterococcus, Klebsiella, and Enterobacter (Csendes A, 1996).

There are four pathophysiological stages of AC, with a clear-cut chronologic correlation with the onset of symptoms: (1) edematous (2–4 days), (2) necrotizing (3–5 days), (3) suppurative (7–10 days), and (4) chronic (Kimura Y, 2007).

During the initial stages of an AC, the connective tissue surrounding the gall bladder is, concurrently, both edematous and hyperemic, a factor that makes dissection easy, albeit with a certain risk of bleeding (Chandler CF, 2000). Later on, with the development of fibrosis and neovascularization, the inflamed tissues retract, making dissection a potentially more difficult task (Rattner DW, 1993. Lo CM, 1998. Serralta AS, 2003).

Clinical Picture and Diagnosis

The typical clinical picture of an attack of AC is that of acute lasting pain in the right hypochondrium, and epigastrium with a positive Murphy sign (specificity 67%–96%) associated with fever, and, in some cases, loss of appetite, nausea, and vomiting (Barbara L, 1987. Kraag N, 1995).

Laboratory studies invariably show leukocytosis with, less frequently, elevation of bilirubin, transaminases, and amylase (Kurzweil SM, 1994).

Abdominal ultrasound is the most conclusive imaging study in case of a suspected diagnosis of AC. Its sensitivity and specificity are higher than 90% (Cooperberg PL, 1980. Ralls PW, 1985. Shea JA, 1994. Chatziioannou SN, 2000. Kalimi R, 2001. Trowdridge RL, 2003. Kiewiet JJ, 2012). The usual diagnostic findings are the presence of gallstones in association with thickening of the gall bladder wall (more than 4 mm), and a sonographically positive Murphy's sign.

The sensitivity of magnetic resonance cholangiography for detecting gall bladder wall thickening is around 69%, being mainly indicated in cases of suspected stones in the biliary tree, where its sensitivity approaches 100% (Parks MS, 1998).

Computed tomography is not routinely indicated for the diagnosis of AC, mainly because of the high false negative figures for the detection of gallstones. It can prove useful in screening for complications or in the differential diagnosis (Barakos JA, 1987. Benarroch-Gampel J, 2011).

Treatment

The therapeutic management of AC dictates admission to an acute surgical bed for adequate fluid and electrolyte support, as well as the administration of analgesics. The use of antibiotics is not well-defined in non-complicated cases, bearing in mind that AC is primarily an inflammatory pathology without infection in the majority of cases (Solomkin JS, 2008). In fact, antibiotic treatment does not seem to alter the course or the recovery of the majority of cases of mild AC (Mazeh H, 2012). Nevertheless, the administration of antibiotics is the usual practice in avoiding the development of septic complications (Javinen HJ, 1978). According to the "Spanish Consensus for Antimicrobial Therapy of Intra-abdominal Infection," and the "Guidelines by the Surgical Infection Society and the Infectious Diseases Society of America," the usual antibiotics employed in AC should be a third generation cephalosporin, in combination with metronidazole, piperacillin-tazobactam, or ertapenem (Imipenem or meropenem in high risk), and, in case of beta-lactam allergy, aztreonam, ciprofloxacin, or gentamicin in combination with metronidazole or clindamycin (Guirao X, 2009. Solomkin JS, 2010). It has been demonstrated that prolonging antibiotic treatment beyond 4 days in patients subjected to EC for moderate AC does not reduce the risk of surgical site infection (Rodríguez-Sanjuán JC, 2013. Regimbeau JM, 2014).

Many authors believe that percutaneous drainage of the gall bladder (Radder RW, 1980. Thistle JL, 1984. Garber SJ, 1994. VanSonnenberg E, 1992. Gervais DA, 1996. Hultman SC, 1996. Patterson EJ, 1996. Van Overhagen H, 1996) or endoscopic transpapillary drainage (Kjaer DW, 2007. Itoi T, 2008) can be considered in high-risk patients (ASA III and IV) and in patients whose diagnosis has been delayed beyond 72 hours. On the other hand, recent publications have demonstrated that cholecystostomy offers little advantage over emergent cholecystectomy, and should be indicated only in very high-risk surgical patients, in whom emergency surgery is absolutely contraindicated (Nahrwold DL, 1976. Kallo AN, 2001. Rodríguez-Sanjuán JC, 2012. Gurusamy KS, 2013). Once recovered from the acute episode, the majority of these patients should undergo elective surgery to remove the gall bladder whenever feasible (Morse BC, 2010).

As mentioned previously, there are two surgical therapeutic options for the treatment of an acute episode of cholecystitis: EC during the same index admission or DC during a later scheduled admission.

The Tokyo Consensus Meeting of 2007 (Yamashita Y, 2007), revised in 2012 (Yokoe M, 2012) and 2013 (Takada T, 2013), established guidelines for the management of AC, including diagnostic criteria (Table 1) and severity criteria (Table 2), as well as treatment schemes (Figure 3).

Table 1. Diagnostic criteria for acute cholecystitis

(1) Murphy's sign, (2) RUQ mass/pain/tenderness
B. Systemic signs of inflammation, etc.:
(1) Fever, (2) elevated CRP, (3) abnormal WBC count
C. Imaging findings: imaging findings characteristic of acute cholecystitis
DEFINITE DIAGNOSIS
(1) One item in A + one item in B are positive
(2) C confirms the diagnosis when acute cholecystitis is suspected clinically

Acute hepatitis, other acute abdominal diseases, and chronic cholecystitis should be excluded.

WBC: white blood cell RUQ: right upper quadrant CRP: C-reactive protein.

Table 2. Severity assessment criteria for acute cholecystitis

"Severe" (Grade III) acute cholecystitis is accompanied by dysfunctions in any one of the following organs/systems:	
1. Cardiovascular dysfunction	Hypotension requiring treatment with dopamine $\geq$5 μg/kg per min, or any dose of dobutamine
2. Neurological dysfunction	Decreased level of consciousness
3. Respiratory dysfunction	PaO_2/FiO_2 ratio <300
4. Renal dysfunction	Oliguria, creatinine >2.0 mg/dl
5. Hepatic dysfunction	PT-INR >1.5
6. Hematological dysfunction	Platelet count <100,000/mm^3
"Moderate" (Grade II) acute cholecystitis is accompanied by any one of the following conditions:	
1. Elevated WBC count (>18,000/mm^3)	
2. Palpable tender mass in the right upper abdominal quadrant	
3. Duration of complaints >72 h	
4. Marked local inflammation (gangrenous cholecystitis, pericholecystic abscess, hepatic abscess, biliary peritonitis, emphysematous cholecystitis)	
"Mild" (Grade I) acute cholecystitis does not meet the criteria of "Severe (Grade III)" or "Moderate (Grade II)" acute cholecystitis. Grade I can also be defined as acute cholecystitis in a healthy patient with no organ dysfunction and only mild inflammatory changes in the gallbladder, making cholecystectomy a safe and low-risk operative procedure.	

WBC: white blood cell.

Table 3. Comparative table of results

		Morbidity	B.leakage	Major injury	Infection	Bleeding	Mort.	Conv.	Stay
V. Linden	EC	14.3%	0%		12.9%		0%		10.1
	DC				1.7%				19.9
Lo	EC	13%	0%				0%	11%	6
	DC	29%						24%	
Johanson	EC	19%	8%	0%	3%	8%		31%	5
	DC	10%	0%	1%	4%	1%		29%	8
Papi	EC						0.2%		7-10
	DC						0.9%		20.4
Gurusamy	EC	6.5% (SEVERE)	3.2%	0.4%				20.3%	4-8
	DC	5% (SEVERE)	0%	0.9-1.4%				23.6%	8-12
Gutt	EC	11.6	1%	0.3%					
	DC	31.3	0.3%	0.3%					
Menahem	EC	14.7%	2.4%	0.8%				13.9%	5.4
	DC	21.4%	0.3%	0.9%				13.9%	9.1
Authors	EC	25.9%	2.2%	0.57%	8.6%	2.3%	1.1%	22%	8.3
	DC	28%	3.6%	0.97%	2.3%	0%	3.5%	19%	12.9

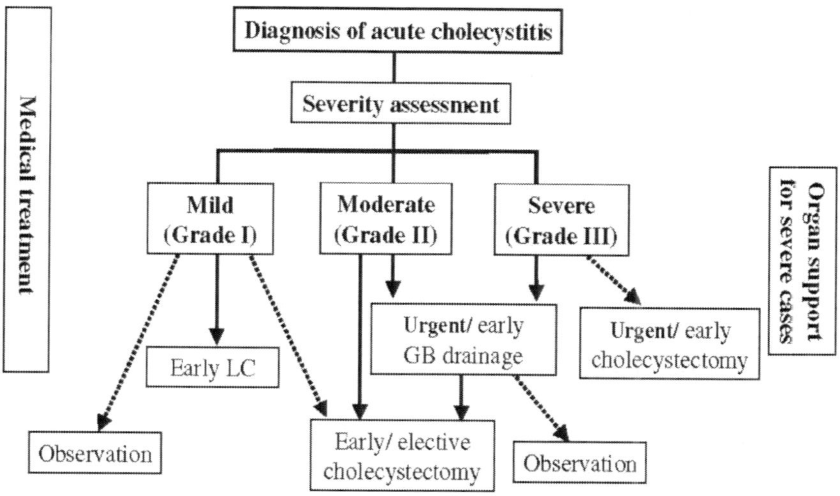

Figure 1. Flowchart for the management of acute cholecystitis.

Early Cholecystectomy and Delayed Cholecystectomy in the Treatment of Acute Cholecystitis

The first studies that assessed EC as a treatment option for AC date back to the fifties (Ellison EH, 1957. Mulholland JH, 1957. Pines B, 1959). In 1970, Van der Linden published the first controlled study demonstrating better morbidity and average hospital stay after open EC (Van der Linden W, 1970). The exponential development of laparoscopic surgery during the 1990's brought to light the first publications about laparoscopic EC, showing poor results in terms of morbidity and mortality and high percentages of bile duct injuries. Based on these results, laparoscopic EC was abandoned and even considered a contraindication for the treatment of acute cholecystitis, favoring initial conservative treatment followed by a laparoscopic DC.

In 1998, Kiviluoto reported similar results when comparing laparoscopic EC and open EC in terms of morbi-mortality (Kiviluoto T, 1998). That same year, Lo presented the first controlled trial comparing laparoscopic EC and laparoscopic DC with lower morbidity and hospital stay figures in the EC group (Lo CM, 1998). Many authors have reported similar results in favor of laparoscopic EC (Lai PB, 1998. Chandler CF, 2000. Johansson M, 2003. Serralta AS, 2003. Kolla SB, 2004. Gurusamy KS, 2006. Siddiqui T, 2008.

Gurusamy KS, 2010. Banz V, 2011. Gurusamy KS, 2013. Gutt CN, 2013. Menahem B, 2015). It is important to note that the vast majority of the recent publications only include laparoscopic cases, which could cause a bias in the external validity of these studies as they may exclude many of the less favorable cases managed by open EC.

In spite of the wealth of publications in favor of EC, there is still controversy regarding the optimal timing to perform a cholecystectomy in the acute situation. Although the literature favors laparoscopic EC, most evidence is based on prospective studies specifically designed to prove this particular point (Lai PB, 1998. Lo CM, 1998. Chandler CF, 2000. Johansson M, 2003. Serralta AS, 2003. Kolla SB, 2004. Gurusamy KS, 2006), which probably does not reflect the worldwide clinical practice, whereby laparoscopic EC is not the rule in most hospitals (Feliu X, 2003. Senapati PS, 2003. Vetrhus M, 2003. Livingston EH, 2004. Papi C, 2004. Shikata S, 2005. Gurusamy KS, 2006. Gutt CN, 2013).

DEFINITIONS

DC is defined as an elective operation, performed after successful conservative management of an acute episode of cholecystitis. Usually, the waiting period between both admissions is in the range of 6–8 weeks. A shortening of this interval could result in an operation during the subacute inflammatory process, while waiting too long could increase the risk of readmissions and complications. Cholecystectomies performed after 72 hours from the onset of symptoms have been considered as delayed surgery in some studies (González-Rodríguez F, 2009. Chandler CF, 2000).

All the publications about DC show a proportion of patients in whom conservative management has failed and an operation had to be performed urgently or earlier than expected. The figures of urgent cholecystectomy during the index admission oscillate between 18% and 38% for some authors (Senapati PS, 2003. Lau H, 2006. Barceló M, 2013. Gurusamy KS, 2013), and around 12% to 13% in other cases (Jarvinen HJ, 1980. Norrby S, 1983). Of note, between 9% and 26% of patients will never be operated for any different reasons (Jarvinen HJ, 1980. Norrby S, 1983. Vetrhus M, 2003. Papi C, 2004. Lau H, 2006. Barceló M, 2013).

The EC concept has undergone various modifications since its inception in the fifties, defined as the surgery performed either during the first 4 days of the acute illness (Pines B, 1959. Dávila D, 1999), during the first 72 hours after the onset of symptoms (Lo CM, 1996), during the first 72 hours after the hospital admission (Lo CM, 1998), during the first 24 hours after admission (Lai PB, 1998. Gutt CN, 2013), during the first 7 days after the onset of symptoms (Johansson M, 2003. Gurusamy KS, 2013. De Mestral C, 2014), or during the first 5 days after admission (Banz V, 2011).

In the present time, the "golden period" consensus defines EC as one that is performed during the first 72 hours after the onset of symptoms (Kimura Y, 2007). Patients submitted to surgery during this golden period suffer less blood loss, lower conversion rates, a shorter hospital stay, and incur lower hospital costs (Rattner DW, 1993. Garber SM, 1997. Eldar S, 1997. Lai PB, 1998. Lo CM, 1998. Chandler CF, 2000. Johansson M, 2003. Serralta AS, 2003). Nevertheless, our own experience and that of other surgeons have shown that delaying surgery due to exceeding of this time period could not be justified, as data for morbi-mortality and conversion rates seem to be comparable for operations performed during the first 72 hours and surgeries performed afterwards (Dobois F, 1990. Kiviluoto T, 1998).

MORBIDITY

Many of the published studies show higher rates of overall morbidity in patients submitted to DC. However, analyzing the morbidity figures of some of the most influential studies demonstrates that there are no significant differences between EC and DC (Papi C, 2004. Gurusamy KS, 2006). The percentage of severe complications (Clavien III-IV) is around 6% in both groups, with slightly higher figures of severe morbidity in the EC group (Gurusamy KS, 2013).

Data from our experience indicate that DC has a higher complication rate than EC, mainly due to a higher proportion of minor surgical complications. We observed that the risk of complications is 50% higher in patients with Charlson Index > 3 who underwent DC, but there is no statistically significant difference from patients with Charlson index < 3. We conclude that patients who benefit the most from EC are the elderly with elevated comorbidities (Charlson Index > 3), a fact that has been highlighted in other recent studies (Ferrarese AG, 2003. Rodriguez-Sanjuán JC, 2012. Cheng Y, 2013. Haltmeier T, 2015).

It is important to note that there is a morbidity factor that has not yet been analyzed, which we believe may be of great interest and, in some way, a crucial factor in supporting the EC as the optimal treatment for AC; that factor is the assessment, within the DC group, of the medical complications arising during the medical treatment of cholecystitis and during the waiting period before the elective cholecystectomy, as well as the deterioration in health of the patient occurring between the index episode and the elective cholecystectomy.

Subtotal cholecystectomy could be taken into account in severe cases of AC, because it can prevent serious surgical complications, such as bleeding and bile duct injuries, in both EC and DC.

Surgical Site Infection

From a theoretical point of view, higher rates of post-operative infection in EC would be expected, due to frequent gallbladder infection at the time of surgery.

The comparative results of publications regarding the incidence of surgical site infection are highly variable, and most are found in outdated studies (Van der Linden W, 1970. Lahtinen J, 1978. Jarvinen HJ, 1980. Norrby S, 1983). Gurusamy published a higher percentage of surgical site infection that required percutaneous drainage in the EC group (Gurusamy KS, 2006). On the other hand, in our experience, the risk of postoperative infection is twice as high in the DC group as in the EC one.

Bleeding

As discussed previously, during the initial stages of an AC, the connective tissue surrounding the gall bladder is edematous and hyperemic, which could facilitate dissection, but with a potentially higher risk of bleeding in EC (Chandler CF, 2000).

Accordingly, some authors noted a lower bleeding risk in DC than in EC (Norrby S, 1983. Johansson M, 2003), which concurs with our own results.

Bile Duct Injury

After an initial conservative treatment, with the development of fibrosis and neovascularization, the inflamed tissues retract, making dissection a potentially more difficult task (Rattner DW, 1993. Lo CM, 1998. Serralta AS, 2003), which could involve a higher risk of bile duct injuries.

Many authors do not show significant differences in the proportion of bile duct injury between EC and DC (Gurusamy KS, 2006. Gurusamy KS, 2010. Gurusamy KS 2013. Menahem B, 2015), despite the rate of biliar injury of DC doubling that of the EC in some cases (Gurusamy shows 0.4% of severe lesions in EC, and 0.9% in DC).

MORTALITY

Most studies present similar mortality rates for both groups, with percentages close to 1% (Papi C, 2004. Banz V, 2011), or without mortality or no registered mortality (Gurusamy KS, 2006. Gurusamy KS, 2010. Gurusamy KS 2013).

In our experience, the mortality rate is more than twice as high in the DC group as in the EC group, but the differences were not found to be statistically significant. It is remarkable that the hospital mortality of patients who did not undergo surgery in the DC group is 8.9%, and the mortality of these patients in the first three years after the index episode is 51.1%.

DAYS OF HOSPITAL STAY

All articles published to date have found a significantly lower hospital stay in EC, with differences ranging from 2 days (Banz V, 2011) to 10 days (Van der Linden W, 1970. Papi C, 2004). According to our experience, patients who underwent surgery after 72 hours from the onset of symptoms presented a significantly higher hospital stay than patients operated on within the first 72 hours, due to a longer stay before surgery, a fact pointed out in many other studies (Rattner DW, 1993. Garber SM, 1997. Eldar S, 1997. Lai PB, 1998. Lo CM, 1998. Chandler CF, 2000. Johansson M, 2003. Serralta AS, 2003.

Readmissions

Lahtinen and Lau published readmission figures before elective surgery of between 25% and 30% in the DC group (Lahtinen J, 1978. Lau H, 2006). In our experience, DC has a higher readmission rate (21.9% vs. 6.8%), due to readmissions occurring between the index episode and elective cholecystectomy (18.2%). Furthermore, readmission rates are twice as high among non-operated patients within the DC group, compared to patients submitted to surgery urgently or electively.

Admission to Intensive Care Unit

No information in relation to the admission to ICU was found in the analyzed articles. In our experience, there is a significantly lower rate of ICU admission among patients of the EC group (2.3%) compared to the DC group (7.8%). The high rate of ICU admission (21.7%) among patients requiring urgent surgery in the DC group is remarkable.

Type Of Surgery and Conversion Rates

Nowadays, laparoscopic cholecystectomy, either early or delayed, is considered as safe as the open operation. We do, however, believe that there is insufficient data from well-designed randomized studies, where patients are not selected for the type of surgery according to their age, morbidity, or the severity of their cholecystitis.

In our experience, there is a significantly higher proportion of moderate and severe cases of cholecystitis in patients who were submitted to open surgery. This may involve a questionable external validity of studies that only include the laparoscopic approach, due to dismissal of cases with a potentially worse prognosis.

The conversion rates from laparoscopic to open surgery are very similar in EC and DC, with figures that vary between 15% and 30% in most studies reviewed (Lai PB, 1998. Johansson M, 2003. Kolla SB, 2004. Gurusamy KS, 2013. Gutt CN, 2013). Other authors report lower conversion rates in EC (3–13%) than in DC (17–25%) (Lo CM, 1998. Eldar S, 1999. Serralta AS, 2003. Papi C, 2004).

The risk factors associated with conversion to open surgery are male gender (Bickel A, 1996. Russell JC, 1998), age above 65 (Lo CM, 1996), severity of the inflammatory process, undue delay between the onset of symptoms and surgery (Rattner DW, 1993. Bickel A, 1996. Garber SM, 1997. Eldar S, 1997), gallbladder wall thickness of more than 5 mm (Braghetto I, 1997), large-sized stones (Lo CM, 1997), previous history of biliary disease (Eldar S, 1997), and lack of laparoscopic expertise on the part of the operating surgeon (Rattner DW, 1993. Bickel A, 1996. Bender JS, 2002. Gharaibeh KI, 2002. Rosen M, 2002).

Subtotal cholecystectomy could be a resource for reducing the conversion rate of laparoscopic cholecystectomies in severe cholecystitis cases.

Duration of Surgery

Published meta-analysis does not show remarkable differences between EC and DC regarding the duration of the operative procedure. Nonetheless, some authors have highlighted a shorter duration in the EC group (Lai PB, 1998. Lo CM, 1998. Dávila D, 1999).

Reoperations

Data published by Banz showed a greater percentage of reoperations in the DC group (27.9%) than in EC group (11.9%) (Banz V, 2011). In our experience, the chance of reoperation was almost twice as high in EC (4.6%) than in DC (2.4%), but this ratio was not found to be statistically significant.

Hospital Costs and Time Off Work

Recent studies point out that direct costs of EC treatment are lower than those of DC, highlighting EC as a more cost-effective approach (Wilson E, 2010. Gutt CN, 2013. Johner A, 2013). Furthermore, EC could mean a reduction in time off work (Van der Linden W, 1970. Norrby S, 1983. Gurusamy KS, 2010).

Subtotal Cholecystectomy

Subtotal cholecystectomy for severe AC could be an alternative that helps avoid serious complications and laparotomies, both in EC and DC, whenever safe dissection of the Calot's triangle is not feasible. There are two types of subtotal cholecystectomy, namely the "fenestrating" and the "reconstituting." Subtotal reconstituting cholecystectomy closes off the lower end of the gall bladder, thereby reducing the risk of postoperative fistula, but creates a remnant gallbladder, which may result in the recurrence of symptoms. Subtotal fenestrating cholecystectomy does not occlude the gallbladder, but may suture the cystic duct internally. It has a higher incidence of postoperative biliary fistula, but does not appear to be associated with recurrent gallstones.

The vast majority of subtotal cholecystectomies are performed in severe cases of AC (80%). Other indications include patients with liver cirrhosis, Mirizzi syndrome, or in cases of anatomic uncertainty. The morbidity and mortality figures are similar to those of total cholecystectomy. However, the subtotal operation reduces the risk of biliary injury to almost zero, while increasing the possibility of bile leaks.

Laparoscopic subtotal cholecystectomy is feasible and safe, offering the advantage of avoiding a laparotomy; however, it requires advanced laparoscopic skills. (Rohatgi A, 2006. Kaplan D, 2014. Elshaer M, 2015. Shingu Y, 2016. Strasberg SM, 2016).

Is Delayed Cholecystectomy for Acute Cholecystitis Indicated in Some Clinical Situations?

While EC seems to be the most appropriate treatment for AC, the choice of an initial conservative treatment, associated or not with cholecystostomy, should be taken into account in some specific clinical situations:

- Xanthogranulomatous cholecystitis is a rare but severe presentation of cholecystitis, characterized by extensive inflammation of the gallbladder wall. Frequently, radiological images can lead to suspect the presence of a gallbladder cancer, which complicates therapeutic decisions (Ladefoged C, 1993. Psarras K, 2012. Cui Y, 2013).

- The treatment approach of AC during pregnancy is a delicate situation for any surgeon. Non-surgical management seems to be associated with a higher incidence of spontaneous abortion, threatened abortion, and premature birth, in addition to recurrent symptoms and more emergency department visits, when compared to patients who underwent cholecystectomy (Curet MJ, 2000. Othman MO, 2012). Laparoscopy is the recommended approach up to the beginning of the 3rd trimester, and maternal mortality with laparoscopic cholecystectomy is not increased by the pregnancy (Cosenza CA, 1999). On the other hand, initial conservative treatment associated with percutaneous transhepatic gallbladder drainage is a safe procedure to be considered in pregnant women with cholecystitis, in which cholecystectomy is not possible or is associated with an unacceptably high risk (Eller A, 2016).
- The most suitable treatment of AC associated with choledocholithiasis, with or without cholangitis, seems to be ERCP followed by laparoscopic cholecystectomy, provided that the clinical picture does not compel urgent surgery (Internal Clinical Guidelines Team. UK, 2014). Depending on the ERCP timing, cholecystectomy will be early or delayed.
- DC may be the best therapeutic option for AC in some critically ill patients, or in patients with any serious disease where surgery is contraindicated at that time. In these cases, consideration of a cholecystostomy as part of conservative treatment tends to be the rule (Boggi U, 1999. Bitner M, 2013. Gurusamy KS, 2013. Bala M, 2015).

KEY MESSAGES

- The golden period for performing an EC is during the first 72 hours after symptom onset, but delaying surgery when this time limit is exceeded does not appear to be justified in the majority of cases.
- In a DC protocol of management, about 20%-30% of patients will require urgent surgery during the index admission, 10%–30% will be readmitted for recurrent bouts of AC before the scheduled date of their elective surgery, and about 12%–30% will reject the operation after initial management. This means that, in the best scenario, only 50% of the patients will get their elective operation after the index

episode, leaving half of the cases at risk of complications and mortality.

- There is no clear evidence that EC is more beneficial than DC in terms of morbidity and mortality, but there is a clear-cut trend in its favor.
- EC reduces total hospital stay and has a lower readmission rate.
- There is not enough evidence comparing the differences between EC and DC with regards to duration of surgery, conversion rates, admission to ICU, and reoperations. It does seem, however, that there is a clear trend in favor of the EC protocol of management.
- EC seems to lead to a reduction in direct hospital costs, to be more cost-effective, and to shorten the time off work.
- Transhepatic cholecystostomy and trans-cystic biliary drainage can be taken into account as part of the therapeutic options in some specific cases.
- Subtotal cholecystectomy may have the advantage of avoiding bile duct injury, and could decrease the conversions rate in laparoscopic procedures.
- We would recommend DC in cases where choledocholithiasis or gallbladder cancer cannot be ruled out, and in those with an unacceptable anesthetic risk at the time of diagnosis or a very long evolution of the symptoms.

REFERENCES

Bala M, Mizrahi I, Mazeh H, Yuval J, Eid A, Almogy G. Percutaneous cholecystostomy is safe and effective option for acute calculous cholecystitis in select group of high-risk patients. *Eur J Trauma Emerg Surg* 2015 Nov 26.

Banz V, Gsponer T, Candinas D, Güller U. Population-based analysis of 4113 patients with acute cholecystitis. Defining the optimal time-point for laparoscopic cholecystectomy. *Ann Surg* 2011; 00:1-7.

Barakos JA, Ralls PW, Lapin SA, et al. Cholelithiasis: evaluation with CT. *Radiology* 1987; 162:415.

Barbara L, Sama C, Morselli AM, et al. A population study on the prevalence of gallstone disease: the Sirmione Study. *Hepatology* 1987; 7:913.

Barceló M, Cruz-Santamaría DM, Alba-López C, Devesa-Medina MJ, Díaz-Rubio M, Rey E. Advantages of early cholecystectomy in clinical practice of a terciary care center. *Hepatobiliary Pancreat Dis Int* 2013; 12(1):87-93.

Bateson MC. Gallbladder disease and Cholecistectomy rates are independently variable. *Lancet* 1984; 2:621-624.

Benarroch-Gampel J, Boyd CA, Sheffield KM, et al. Overuse of CT in patients with complicated gallstone disease. *J Am Coll Surg* 2011; 213:524.

Bender JS, Duncan MD, Freeswick PD, Harmon JW, Magnuson TH. Increased laparoscopic experience does not lead to improved results with acute cholecystitis. *Am J Surg* 2002; 184:591-5.

Bickel A, Rappaport A, Kanlevski V, Haj M, Geron N, Eitan A. Laparoscopic management of acute cholecystitis: prognostic factors for success. *Surg Endosc* 1996; 10:1045.

Bitner M, Jaszewski R, Jander S, Maciejewski M. Laparoscopic cholecystectomy delayed by complicated myocardial infarction with papillary muscle rupture, and performed after unique complex mitral repair. *Wideochir Inne Tech Maloinwazyjne* 2013 Jun;8(2):170-3.

Boggi U, Di Candio G, Campatelli A, Oleggini M, Pietrabissa A, Filipponi F, Bellini R, Mazzotta D, Mosca F. Percutaneous cholecystostomy for acute cholecystitis in critically ill patients. *Hepatogastroenterology* 1999 Jan-Feb;46(25):121-5.

Braghetto I, Csendes A, Debandi A, Korn O, Bastias J. Correlation among ultrasonographic and videoscopic findings of the gallbladder: surgical difficulties and reasons for conversion during laparoscopic surgery. *Surg Laparosc Endosc* 1997; 7:310.

Chandler CF, Lane JS, Ferguson P, Thomson JE, Ashley SW. Prospective evaluation of early versus delayed laparoscopic cholecystectomy for treatment of acute cholecystitis. *Am Surg* 2000; 66:896-900.

Chatziioannou SN, Moore WH, Ford PV, Dhekne RD. Hepatobiliary scintygraphy is superior to abdominal ultrasonography in suspected acute cholecystitis. *Surgery* 2000; 127:609.

Cheng Y, Leng J, Tan J, Chen K, Dong J. Proper surgical technique approved for early laparoscopic Cholecystectomy for non-critically ill elderly patients with acute cholecystitis. *Hepatogastroenterology* 2013; 60(124):688-91.

Cooperberg PL, Burhenne HJ. Real-time ultrasonography. Diagnostic technique of choice in calculous gallbladder disease. *N Eng J Med* 1980; 302:1277.

Cosenza CA, Saffari B, Jabbour N, et al. Surgical management of biliary gallstone disease during pregnancy. *Am J Surg* 1999; 178:545-548.

Csendes A, Burdiles P, Maluenda F, et al. Simultaneous bacteriologic assessment of bile from gallbladder and common bile duct in control subjets and patients with gallstones and common duct stones. *Arch Surg* 1996; 131:389.

Cui Y, Zhang H, Zhao E, Cui N, Li Z. Differential diagnosis and treatment options for xanthogranulomatous cholecystitis. *Med Princ Pract* 2013;22(1):18-23.

Curet MJ. Special problems in laparoscopic surgery. Previous abdominal surgery, obesity, and pregnancy. *Surg Clin North Am* 2000; 80:1093-1110.

Dávila D, Manzanares C, Pincho ML, Albors P, Cardenas F, Fuster E, et al. Experience in the treatment (early vs. Delayed) of acute cholecystitis via laparoscopy. *Cir Esp* 1999; 66(suppl 1):233.

De Mestral C, Rotstein OD, Laupacis A, Hoch JS, Zagorski B, Alali AS, Nathens AB. Comparative operative outcomes of early and delayed cholecystectomy for acute cholecystitis. A population-based propensity score analysis. *Ann Surg* 2014;259(1):10-15.

Dobois F, Icard P, Berthelot G, et al. Coelioscopic Cholecystectomy: preliminary report of 36 cases. *Ann Surg* 1990; 211:60-2.

Eldar S, Sabo E, Nash E, Abrahamson J, Matter I. Laparoscopic cholecystectomy for acute cholecystitis: prospective trial. *World J Surg* 1997; 21:540-5.

Eldar S, Eitan A, Bickel A, et al. The impact of patient delay and physician delay on the outcome of laparoscopic cholecystectomy for acute cholecystitis. *Am J Surg* 1999; 178:303-7.

Eller A, Shim S, Sigvardt L, Rask P, Nielsen MF. Treatment of acute cholecystitis in a third-trimester pregnant women. *Ugeskr Laeger* 2016 Apr 18;178(16).

Ellison EH, Miholland JH, Friesen SR. Early operation for acute cholecystitis. Current Surgical Management. *Philadelphia, Saunders* 1957.

Elshaer M, Gravante G, Thomas K, Sorge R, Al-Hamali S, Ebdewi H. Subtotal cholecystectomy for "difficult gallbladders": systematic review and meta-analysis. *JAMA Surg* 2015 Feb;150(2):159-68.

Feliu X, Targarona EM, Garcia A, Pey A, et al. La cirugía laparoscópica en España. Resultados de la encuesta nacional de la Sección de Cirugía Endoscópica de la Asociación Española de Cirujanos. *Cir Esp* 2003; 74(3):164-70.

Ferrarese AG, Solej M, Enrico S, Falcone A, Catalano S, Pozzi G, Marola S, Martino V. Elective and emergency laparoscopic cholecystectomy in the elderly: our experience. *BMC surg* 2003; 13 Suppl 2:S21.

Friedman GD, Raviola CA, Fireman B. Prognosis of gallstones with mild or no syntoms: 25 years of follow-up in a health maintenance organization. *J Clin Epidemiol* 1989; 42:127.

Friedman GD. Natural history of asymptomatic and symptomatic gallstones. *Am J Surg* 1993; 165:399.

Garber SJ, Mathleson JR, Coopergerg PL, et al. Percutaneous cholecystostomy: safety of the transperitoneal route. *J Vasc Interv Radiol* 1994; 5:295-8.

Garber SM, Korman J, Cosgrove JM, Cohen JR. Early laparoscopic cholecystectomy for acute cholecystitis. *Surg Endosc* 1997; 11:347-50.

Gervais DA, Mueller PR. Percutaneus cholecystostomy. *Semin Intervent Radiol* 1996;13:35-43.

Gharaibeh KI, Qasaimeh GR, Al-Heiss H, Ammari F Bani-Hani K, Al-jaberi TM, et al. Effects of timing of surgery, type of inflamation and sex on outcome of laparoscopic cholecystectomy for acute cholecystitis. *J Laparoendosc Adv Surg Tech* 2002; 12:193-8.

Guirao X, Arias J, Badía JM, García-Rodríguez JA, Mensa J, Alvarez-Lerma F, Borges M, Barberán J, Maseda E, Salavert M, Llinares P, Gobernado M, García Rey C. Recommendations in the empiric anti-infective agents of intra-abdominal infection. *Rev Esp Quimioter* 2009 Sep;22(3):151-72.

Gurusamy KS, Samraj K. Early versus delayed laparoscopic cholecystectomy for acute cholecystitis (review). *Cochrane Database Syst Rev* 2006; (4):CD005440.

Gurusamy KS, Samraj K, Gluud C, Wilson E, Davidson BR. Meta-analysis of randomized controlled trials on the safety and effectiveness of early versus delayed laparoscopic cholecystectomy for acute cholecystitis. *Br J Surg* 2010; 97(2):141-50.

Gurusamy KS, Davidson C, Gluud C, Davidson BR. Early versus delayed laparoscopic cholecystectomy for people with acute cholecystitis. *Cochrane Database Syst Rev* 2013; 6:CD005440.

Gurusamy KS, Rossi M, Davidson BR. Percutaneous Cholecystostomy for high-risk surgical patients with acute calculous cholecystitis. *Cochrane Database Syst Rev* 2013; 8:CD007088.

Gutt CN, Encke J, Koninger J, Harnoss JC, Weigand K, Kipfmuller K, et al. Acute cholecystitis. Early versus delayed cholecystectomy, a multicenter randomized trial (ACDC study). *Ann Surg* 2013; 258(3):385-93.

Haltmeier T, Benjamin E, Inaba K, Lam M, Demetriades D. Early versus delayed same-admission laparoscopic cholecystectomy for acute cholecystitis in elderly patients with comorbidities. J *Trauma Acute Care Surg* 2015 Mar 4.

Hultman SC, Herbst AC, McCall MC, et al. The efficacy of percutaneous cholecystostomy in critically ill patients. *Am J Surg* 1996; 62:263-9.

Internal Clinical Guidelines Team (UK). Gallstone Disease: Diagnosis and Management of Cholelithiasis, Cholecystitis and Choledocholithiasis. London: National Institute for Health and *Care Excellence (UK)*; 2014 Oct.

Itoi T, Sofuni A, Itokawa F, et al. Endoscopic transpapillary gallbladder drainage in patients with acute cholecystitis in whom percutaneous transhepatic approach is contraindicated or anatomically impossible. *Gastrointest Endosc* 2008; 68:455.

Javinen HJ, Renkonen OV, Palmu A. Antibiotics in acute cholecystitis. *Ann Clin Res* 1978; 10:247.

Jarvinen HJ, Hastbacka J. Early cholecystectomy for acute cholecystitis. A prospective randomized study. *Ann Surg* 1980; 191:501-5.

Johansson M, Thune A, Blomqvist A, et al. Management of acute cholecystitis in the laparoscopic era: results of a prospective, randomized clinical trial. *J Gastrointest Surg* 2003; 7:642-5.

Johner A, Raymakers A, Wiseman SM. Cost utility of early versus delayed laparoscopic cholecystectomy for acute cholecystitis. *Surg Endosc* 2013; 27:256-62.

Kalimi R, Gecelter GR, Caplin D, et al. Diagnosis of acute cholecystitis: sensitivity of sonography, cholescintigraphy and combined sonography-cholescinigraphy. *J AM Coll Surg* 2001; 193:609.

Kallo AN, Kantsevoy SV. Gallstones and biliary disease. Prim Care 2001; 28:591.

Kaplan D, Inaba K, Chouliaras K, Low GM, Benjamin E, Lam L, Grabo D, Demetriades D. Subtotal cholecystectomy and open total cholecystectomy: alternatives in complicated cholecystitis. *Am Surg* 2014 Oct; 80(10):953-5.

Kiewiet JJ, Leeuwenburgh MM, Bipat S, et al. A systematic review and meta-analysis of diagnostic performance of imaging in acute cholecystitis. *Radiology* 2012; 264:708.

Kiviluoto T, Siren J, Luukkonen P, et al. Randomized trial of laparoscopic versus open cholecystectomy for acute and gangrenous cholecystitis. Lancet 1998; 351: 321-5.

Kjaer DW, Kruse A, Funch-Jensen P. Endoscopic gallbladder drainage of patients with acute cholecystitis. *Endoscopy* 2007; 39:304.

Kolla SB, Aggarwal S, Kumar A, Kumar R, Chumber S, Parshad R, et al. Early versus delayed laparoscopic cholecystectomy for acute cholecystitis. *Surg Endosc* 2004; 18:1323-7.

Kraag N, Thijs C, Knipschild P. Dyspepdia: how noisy are gallstones? A meta-analysis of epidemiologic studyes of biliary pain, dyspeptic syntoms and food intolerance. *Scand J Gastroenterol* 1995; 30:411.

Kurzweil SM, Shapiro MJ, Andrus CH, et al. Hyperbilirubinemia without common bile duct abnormalities and hyperamylasemia without pancreatitis in patients with gallbladder disease. *Arch Surg* 1994; 129:829.

Ladefoged C, Lorentzen M. Xanthogranulomatous cholecystitis. A clinicopathological study of 20 cases and review of the literature. *APMIS* 1993 Nov;101(11):869-75.

Lahtinen J, Alhava EM, Aukee S. Acute cholecystitis treated by early and delayed surgery. A controled clinical trial. *Scand J Gastroenterol* 1978; 13:673-8.

Lai PB, Kwong KH, Leung KL, Kwok SP, Chan AC, Chung SC, Lau WY. Randomized trial of early versus delayed laparoscopic cholecystectomy in acute cholecystitis. *Br J Surg* 1998; 85:764-7.

Lau H, Lo CY, Patil NG, Yuen WK. Early versus delayed-interval laparoscopic cholecystectomy for acute cholecystitis. *Surg Endosc* 2006; 20:82-87.

Livingston EH, Rege RV. A nationwide study of conversion from laparoscopic to open cholecystectomy. *Am J Surg* 2004; 188(3):205-11.

Lo CM, Lai EC, Fan ST, Liu CL, Wong J. Laparoscopic cholecystectomy for acute cholecystitis in the elderly. *World J Surg* 1996; 20:983.

Lo CM, Liu CL, Fan ST, Lai EC, et al. Early versus delayed laparoscopic cholecystectomy for treatment of acute cholecystitis. *Ann Surg* 1996; 223:37-42.

Lo CM, Fan ST, Liu CL, et al. Early decision for conversion of laparoscopic to open cholecystectomy for treatment of acute cholecystitis. *Am J Surg* 1997; 173:513-7.

Lo CM, Liu CL, Fan ST, Lai EC, Wong J. Prospective randomized study of early versus delayed laparoscopic cholecystectomy for acute cholecystitis. *Ann Surg* 1998; 227:461-7.

Mazeh H, Mizrahi I, Dior U, et al. Role of Antibiotic Therapy in Mild Acute Calculus Cholecystitis: A Prospective Randomized Controlled Trial. *World J Surg* 2012; 36(8):1750-9.

Menahem B, Mulliri A, Fohlen A, Guittet L, Alves A, Lubrano J. Delayed laparoscopic cholecystectomy increases the total hospital stay compared to an early laparoscopic cholecystectomy after acute cholecystitis: an updated meta-analysis of randomized controlled trials. *HPB (Oxford)* 2015; 17(10):857-62.

Morris CR, Hohf RP, Ivy AC. An experimental study of the role of stasis in the etiology of cholecystitis. *Surgery* 1952; 32:673.

Morse BC, Smith JB, Lawdahl RB, Roettger RH. Management of acute cholecystitis in critically ill patients: contemporary role for cholecystostomy and subsequent cholecystectomy. *Am Surg* 2010; 76:708.

Mulholland JH, Ellison EH, Friesen SR. Delayed operative management of acute cholecystitis. Current Surgical Management. *Philadelphia, Saunders* 1957.

Nahrwold DL, Rose RC, Ward SP. Abnormalities in gallbladder morphology and function in patients with cholelithiasis. *Ann Surg* 1976; 184:415.

Norrby S, Herlin P, Holmin T, Sjodahl R, Tagesson C. Early or delayed cholecystectomy in acute cholecystitis? A clinical trial. *Br J Surg* 1983; 70:163-5.

Othman MO, Stone E, Hashimi M, Parasher G. Conservative management of cholelithiasis and its complications in pregnancy is associated with recurrent symptoms and more emergency department visits. *Gastrointest Endosc* 2012 Sep;76(3):564-9.

Papi C, Catarci M, Ambrosio D, Gili L, Koch M, Grassi GB, et al. Timing of cholecystectomy for acute calculous cholecystitis: a meta-analysis. *Am J Gastroenterol* 2004; 99(1):147-55.

Parks MS, Yu JS, Kim YH, et al. Acute cholecystitis: comparison of MR cholangiography and US. *Radiology* 1998; 209:781.

Patterson EJ, McLoughlin RF, Mathieson JR, et al. An alternative approach to acute cholecystitis: percutaneous cholecystostomy and interval laparoscopic cholecystectomy. *Surg Endosc* 1996;10:1185-8.

Pines B, Rabinowitch J. Perforation of the gallbladder in acute cholecystitis. *Ann Surg* 1959; 140:170.

Psarras K, Baltatzis ME, Symeonidis N, Pavlidis ET, Miha A, Pavlidis TE, Sakantamis AK. A severe case of xanthogranulomatous cholecystitis along with a review of CT indications for nonoperative management including percutaneous drainage. *Surg Laparosc Endosc Percutan Tech* 2012 Feb;22(1):e42-4.

Radder RW. Ultrasonically guided percutaneous catheter drainage for gallbladder empiema. *Diagn Imaging* 1980; 49:330-3.

Ralls PW, Colleti PM, Lapin SA, et al. Real-time sonography in suspected acute cholecystitis. Prospective evaluation of primary and secondary sings. *Radiology* 1985; 155:767.

Ransohoff DF, Gracie WA. Treatment of gallstones. *Ann Intern Med* 1993; 119:606-19.

Rattner DW, Ferguson C, Warshaw AL. Factors associated with successful laparoscopic cholecystectomy for acute cholecystitis. *Ann Surg* 1993; 217:233-6.

Regimbeau JM, Fuks D, Pautrat K, Mauvais F, Haccart V, Msika S, Mathonnet M, Scotté M, Paquet JC, Vons C, Sielezneff I, Millat B, Chiche L, Dupont H, Duhaut P, Cossé C, Diouf M, Pocard M. Effect of Postoperative Antibiotic Administration on Postoperative Infection Following Cholecystectomy for Acute Calculous Cholecystitis. A Randomized Clinical Trial. *JAMA* 2014;312(2):145-154.

Rodriguez-Sanjuán JC, Arruabarrena A, Sánchez-Moreno L, González-Sánchez F, Herrera LA, Gómez-Fleitas M. Acute cholecystitis in high surgical risk patients: percutaneous cholecystostomy or emergency cholecystectomy?. *Am J Surg* 2012; 204:54-9.

Rodríguez-Sanjuán JC, Casella G, Antolín F, Castillo F, Fernandez-Santiago R, Riaño M, Herrera LA, Gómez-Fleitas. How long is antibiotic theraphy neccesary after urgent cholecystectomy for acute cholecystitis?. *J Gastrointest Surg* 2013; 17(11):1947-52.

Rohatgi A, Singh KK. Mirizzi syndrome: laparoscopic management by subtotal cholecystectomy. *Surg Endosc* 2006 Sep;20(9):1477-81.

Rosen M, Brody F, Ponsky J. Predictive factors for conversion of laparoscopic cholecystectomy. *Am J Surg* 2002; 184:254-8.

Roslyn JJ, DenBesten L, Thomson JE Jr, Silverman BF. Roles of lithogenic bile and cystic duct occlusion in the pathogenesis of acute cholecystitis. *Am J Surg* 1980; 140:126.

Russell JC, Walsh SJ, Reed-Fourquet L, Mattie A, Lynch J. Symptomatic cholelithiasis: a different disease in men?. *Ann Surg* 1988; 227:195.

Senapati PS, Bhattarcharya D, Harinath G, Ammori BJ. A survey of the timing and approach to the surgical management of cholelithiasis in patients with acute biliary pancreatitis and acute cholecystitis in the UK. *Ann R Coll Surg Engl* 2003; 85:306-12.

Serralta AS, Bueno JL, Planells MR, Rodero DR. Prospective evaluation of emergency versus delayed laparoscopic cholecystectomy for early cholecystitis. *Surg Laparosc Endosc Percutan Tech* 2003; 13:71-5.

Shea JA, Berlin JA, Escarce JJ, et al. Revised estimates of diagnostic test sensitivity and specificity in suspected biliary tract disease. *Arch Intern Med* 1994; 154:2573.

Shikata S, Noguchi Y, Fukui T. Early versus delayed cholecystectomy for acute cholecystitis: a meta-analysis of randomized controled trials. *Surg Today* 2005; 35:553-60.

Shingu Y, Komatsu S, Norimizu S, Taguchi Y, Sakamoto E. Laparoscopic subtotal cholecystectomy for severe cholecystitis. *Surg Endosc* 2016 Feb;30(2):526-31.

Siddiqui T, McDonald A, Chong PS, Jenkins JT. Early versus delayed laparoscopic cholecystectomy for acute cholecystitis: a meta-analysisi of randomized clinical trials. *Am J Surg* 2008; 195:40-7.

Solomkin JS, Mazuski JE, Bradley JS, et al. Diagnosis and management of complicated intraabdominal infection in adults and children: guidelines by the Surgical Infection Society and the Infectious Diseases Society of America. *Acad Emerg Med* 2008; 15:718.

Solomkin JS, Mazuski JE, Bradley JS, Rodvold KA, Goldstein EJ, Baron EJ, O'Neill PJ, Chow AW, Dellinger EP, Eachempati SR, Gorbach S, Hilfiker M, May AK, Nathens AB, Sawyer RG, Bartlett JG. Diagnosis and management of complicated intra-abdominal infection in adults and children: guidelines by the Surgical Infection Society and the Infectious Diseases Society of America. *Surg Infect (Larchmt)* 2010 Feb;11(1):79-109.

Strasberg SM, Pucci MJ, Brunt LM, Deziel DJ. Subtotal Cholecystectomy-"Fenestrating" vs "Reconstituting" Subtypes and the Prevention of Bile Duct Injury: Definition of the Optimal Procedure in Difficult Operative Conditions. *J Am Coll Surg* 2016 Jan;222(1):89-96.

Takada T, Strasberg SM, Solomkin JS, Pitt HA, Gomi H, Yoshida M, Mayumi T, Miura F, Gouma DJ, et al. TG13: Updated Tokyo Guidelines for the management of acute cholangitis and cholecystitis. *J Hepatobiliary Pancreat Sci* 2013; 20(1):1-7.

Thistle JL, Cleary PA, Lachin JM, et al. The natural history of cholelithiasis: the National Cooperative Gallstone Study. *Ann Intern Med* 1984; 101:171.

Trowdridge RL, Rutkowski NK, Shojania KG. Does this patient have cholecystitis?. *JAMA* 2003; 289:80.

Van der Linden W, Sunzel H. Early versus delayed operation for acute cholecystitis. A controlled clinical trial. *Am J Surg* 1970; 120:7-13.

Van Overhagen H, Meyers H, Tilanus HW, et al. Percutaneus cholecystostomy for patients with acute cholecystitis and an increased surgical risk. Cardiovasc *Intervent Radiol* 1996; 19:72-76.

VanSonnenberg E, D'Agostino Hb, Goodacre Bw, et al. Percutaneous gallblader puncture and cholecystostomy: results, complications and caveats for safety. *Radiology* 1992; 183:163-70.

Vetrhus M, Soreide O, Nesvik I, Sodenaa K. Acute cholecystitis: delayed surgery or observation. A randomized clinical trial. *Scand J Gastroenterol* 2003; 38:985-90.

Wilson E, Gurusamy K, Gluud C, Davidson BR. Cost-utility and value-of-information analysis of early versus delayed laparoscopic cholecystectomy for acute cholecystitis. *Br J Surg* 2010; 97:210-9.

Yamashita Y, Takada T, Kawarada Y, Nimura Y, Hirota M, e al. Surgical treatment of patients with acute cholecystitis: Tokio Guidelines. *J Hepatobiliary Pancreat Surg* 2007; 14:91-7.

Yokoe M, Takada T, Strasberg SM, Solomkin JS, Mayumi T, et al. New diagnostic criteria and severity assesment of acute cholecystitis: Tokio Guidelines. *J Hepatobiliary Pancreat Surg* 2012; 19:578-85.

In: Acute Cholecystitis
Editor: Lisa Powell
ISBN: 978-1-63485-744-4

Chapter 5

TOKYO GUIDELINES GRADE II (MODERATE) ACUTE CHOLECYSTITIS: A MANAGEMENT DILEMMA?

Mary Caroline Nally, Benjamin R. Veenstra* and Jose M. Velasco
Rush University Medical Center, Chicago, IL US

ABSTRACT

Acute cholecystitis is a common sequelae of cholelithiasis that is encountered in surgical practices worldwide. It varies in severity, causing minimal discomfort in otherwise healthy individuals to being potentially fatal in the critically ill or those with significant comorbidities. In the US alone, it is estimated 500,000 cholecystectomies are performed per year, with an unknown percentage being done for acute cholecystitis. In Japan, the number of cases of acute cholecystitis in a nearly 15 year period had increased from 3.9 million to over 10 million.

Despite being a common and increasingly surgical problem, prior to ten years ago there were no accepted standards for the diagnostic criteria, severity assessment, or management of acute cholecystitis. In 2006, an International Consensus Meeting took place in Tokyo, Japan, where international experts in the field combined personal expertise with evidence based data to create the Tokyo Guidelines, with a revision

* Corresponding author: 1725 W. Harrison St. Suite 810/818 Chicago, IL 60612, Email: Benjamin_Veenstra@Rush.edu.

following in 2013. These guidelines not only assist in making a diagnosis, but provide an algorithm for the management of acute cholecystitis based on severity, or a determined grade. This grade is formulated based upon presenting symptoms, clinical picture, laboratory values, and imaging results. Grade I (mild) acute cholecystitis describes patients with limited or early gallbladder disease and no organ dysfunction. Grade II (moderate) acute cholecystitis describes patients with extensive gallbladder disease and no organ dysfunction. Finally, Grade III (severe) acute cholecystitis describes patients with extensive gallbladder disease and organ dysfunction.

Although cholecystectomy has been the standard of care for the management of acute cholecystitis, the timing, approach, and necessity of a drainage procedure have all have been at the forefront of academic contention. With the introduction and adoption of the Tokyo Guidelines, one would expect these "controversies" to come to rest. While the majority of cases fall into Grade I or III (75%), it is the remaining 25% that prompt a detailed examination of the literature regarding optimal management. For grades I and III acute cholecystitis, management is well established, with laparoscopic cholecystectomy for grade I and antibiotics with early drainage for grade III. On the contrary, Grade II or moderate acute cholecystitis, poses the greatest management dilemma, as its clinical presentation allows for the most variability. In this chapter we examine the current literature as it pertains to the management of patients who present with Grade II (moderate) acute cholecystitis, specifically looking at the timing of operation and the appropriateness of drainage procedures.

Keywords: cholecystitis, Tokyo guidelines, grade II, cholecystostomy, cholecystectomy

INTRODUCTION

Acute cholecystitis is caused by an obstruction in the gallbladder neck or cystic duct leading to obstruction, bile stasis, inflammatory mediator activation, and mucosal injury [1]. Etiologies include gallstones, ischemia, motility disorders, direct chemical injury, microorganism infections, collagen disease, and allergic reaction [1]. Nearly 15% of people in developed countries have gallstones. In the United States, more than 20 million individuals are affected by gallbladder disease each year. One to three percent of those with gallstones develop significant sequelae, such as acute cholangitis or acute cholecystitis [2, 3]. Although mortality is rare, the treatment of gallstone disease is estimated to cost $5.8 billion annually in the United States alone [4]. Thus, the sheer volume and incidence of gallbladder disease, on top of its significant cost burden, make it a relevant topic in healthcare today.

Acute cholecystitis manifests with right upper quadrant pain and fever [5]. Murphy's sign, or cessation of inspiration with inspiration during palpation of the right upper quadrant, is the characteristic physical exam finding of acute cholecystitis [5]. As the presentation of cholecystitis can vary amongst patients, Strasberg concluded that the gold standard for the diagnosis of acute cholecystitis lies in the histopathology of the gallbladder [6]. This is a limited diagnostic tool as histopathology is only available after the specimen has been surgically removed.

Traditionally, there has been little high level evidence for determining the diagnosis or severity of biliary infections [7]. On top of this, there has been no systematically described practical manual for the management of biliary infections [7]. While many studies have been conducted to evaluate the accuracy of diagnostic tests and effectiveness of treatments for this disease process, there has been a significant lag time between the accumulation of such scientific knowledge and its application into clinical practice [4]. To confound matters, more than a dozen *different* diagnostic criteria have historically been used [4]. All of these factors have made it difficult to compare the treatment effectiveness described in studies to actual clinical outcomes across institutions [4].

An example of this lies in the fact that some institutions still use Charcot's triad (abdominal pain, fever, and jaundice) to diagnose cholangitis. However, only 50-70% of patients with acute cholangitis have all three of these clinical findings [3, 7]. These criteria were proposed over 100 years ago, in 1877 and represent level 4 evidence (according to the Oxford Centre for Evidence Based Medicine Levels of Evidence) [7]. Furthermore, severity of acute biliary disease infections also lacks a uniform grading system. Specifically, Reynolds' pentad (abdominal pain, fever, jaundice, shock, decreased consciousness) has been historically used to define patients with severe acute cholangitis [3]. The constellation of these findings is quite rare, being found in only 10% of patients with severe disease [3]. This example illustrates the need for an agreed upon system regarding the diagnosis, classification, and management of biliary infections and pathology.

TOKYO GUIDELINES

Summary

In response to the paucity of a universal definition and management algorithm pertaining to biliary infections, the Committee on the Development of Guidelines for the Management of Acute Biliary Infection prepared "Evidence-based clinical practice guidelines for the management of acute cholangitis and cholecystitis" [3]. The Committee consisted of 46 experts in gastroenterology, surgery, internal medicine, emergency medicine, intensive care, and clinical epidemiology [7]. They were able to finalize a draft of recommendations, which was discussed during four forums by the working group participants as well as an external assessment committee comprised of international leaders in hepatobiliary medicine [7]. This committee met in 2006, reaching a consensus and publishing what has become known as the Tokyo Guidelines in 2007.

First and foremost, the Tokyo Guidelines established the diagnostic criteria for acute cholecystitis. These include 1) local signs of inflammation (Murphy's sign, right upper quadrant mass/pain/tenderness), 2) systemic signs of inflammation (fever, elevated CRP, elevated WBC count), and 3) imaging findings of acute cholecystitis (such as pericholecystic fluid, thickened gallbladder wall, enlarged gallbladder, incarcerated gallstone) [8]. Imaging studies discussed included ultrasonography, MRI, CT, and HIDA scan [8]. A *suspected* diagnosis of acute cholecystitis requires one local sign of inflammation *plus* one systemic sign of inflammation [8]. A diagnosis of acute cholecystitis is *definite* if a patient has one local sign of inflammation *plus* one systemic sign of inflammation *plus* suspicious imaging findings [8]. See Table 1, 2.

Table 1. Diagnostic Criteria for Acute Cholecystitis

Signs of Local Inflammation	Murphy's sign RUQ mass/pain/tenderness
Signs of Systemic Inflammation	Fever Elevated CRP Elevated WBC
Imaging Findings	Imaging findings characteristic of acute cholecystitis

Table 2. Imaging Findings of Acute Cholecystitis

Ultrasonography	Sonographic Murphy sign Thickened gallbladder wall (>4mm) Enlarged gallbladder Incarcerated gallstone, debris echo, pericholecystic fluid Sonolucent layer in the gallbladder wall
MRI	Pericholecystic high signal Enlarged gallbladder Thickened gallbladder wall
CT	Thickened gallbladder wall Pericholecystic fluid collection Enlarged gallbladder Linear high density areas in the pericholecystic fat tissue
Tc-HIDA scan	Non visualized gallbladder with normal uptake and excretion of radioactivity Rim sign (augmentation of radioactivity around the gallbladder fossa)

Beyond providing diagnostic criteria, the Guidelines also established a grading system/assessment of severity, with the hopes to further guide the clinical management of acute cholecystitis. Given there is such a wide spectrum of disease severity at the time of presentation in patients with cholecystitis, a single uniform treatment plan simply is not appropriate. It was proposed that the variability of presentation of acute cholecystitis warrants an individualized treatment algorithm based upon a predefined severity. Thus, the Tokyo Guidelines groups patients with acute cholecystitis into three presenting severity groups. Grade I, or mild acute cholecystitis, is defined as mild gallbladder inflammatory changes in a healthy patient with no organ dysfunction [8]. These patients may be observed with medical therapy or treated with early laparoscopic cholecystectomy. Grade II, or moderate acute cholecystitis, is reserved for patients with any of the following: 1) elevated white blood cell count over 18000/mm3, 2) palpable tender mass in the right upper quadrant, 3) symptoms for more than 72 hours, or 4) marked local inflammation such as abscess, gangrene, emphysema [8]. Given this group has the most variability in presentation; it is not surprising the treatment options are also diverse. These patients may undergo medical therapy, cholecystectomy or gallbladder drainage. Finally, Grade III, or severe acute cholecystitis, is seen in those with organ dysfunction involving the cardiovascular, neurologic, respiratory, renal, hepatic, or hematologic systems

[8]. Due to the systemic effects of biliary disease, these patients are at high risk for operative intervention. Although some may still be appropriate for cholecystectomy, it is recommended that most undergo gallbladder drainage in conjunction with medical therapy (antibiotic treatment). See Table 3.

Table 3. Tokyo Guideline Severity Grades

Mild (Grade I)	Acute cholecystitis in healthy patient with no organ dysfunction and mild inflammatory changes in the gallbladder
Moderate (Grade II)	One of the following: 1) Elevated WBC count (>18,000 mm3) 2) Palpable tender mass in the right upper abdominal quadrant 3) Duration of complaints >72 hours 4) Marked local inflammation (biliary peritonitis, pericholecystic abscess, hepatic abscess, gangrenous cholecystitis, emphysematous cholecystitis)
Severe (Grade III)	One of the following organ dysfunction: 1) Cardiovascular dysfunction (hypotension requiring pressors) 2) Neurological dysfunction (decreased level of consciousness) 3) Respiratory dysfunction (PaO2/FiO2 ratio <300) 4) Renal dysfunction (oliguria, creatine >2mg/dl) 5) Hepatic dysfunction (INR>1.5) 6) Hematological dysfunction (platelets <100,000mm3)

Literature Review

Since the Tokyo Guidelines were released for the diagnosis, severity, and management of acute cholecystitis in 2007, they have been internationally implemented to varying degrees. Revisions were made to the Guidelines in 2013, specifically providing more detailed recommendations for the utilization of imaging findings in diagnosing and grading acute cholecystitis [9]. Given the Tokyo Guidelines were primarily written based on the opinion of experts, it should come as no surprise that several validation studies have been performed, both internationally and within the United States. There have also been an increasing number of studies reviewing current utilization patterns, as well as examining outcomes when these Guidelines are implemented. Here we present and highlight the growing body of literature that evaluates the effectiveness and utility of the Tokyo Guidelines in the clinical arena.

Immediately following the release of the initial Tokyo Guidelines in 2007, Lee et al. performed a retrospective review to assess the potential benefit of implementing the Guidelines into practice [10]. Patients admitted with calculous cholecystitis were identified and then assigned a severity grade using the Tokyo Guidelines. They were then classified into subgroups based on whether their actual clinical management was compatible or incompatible with that recommended by the Tokyo Guidelines [10]. The outcomes, including mortality rate, complications after surgery, and mean length of stay, were analyzed between the subgroups to assess the impact of the Tokyo Guidelines on management of acute cholecystitis [10]. The study found there was no significant difference in survival, post-surgical complications, or mortality. However, those patients who were managed according to the Tokyo Guidelines were found to have a shorter hospital stay in comparison to those managed independently [10].

The accuracy of the Tokyo Guidelines' pre-operative severity assessment was examined next. Ambe et al. performed a single institution retrospective review over a 5 year period, comparing the pre-operative severity grade of each patient to the extent of gallbladder inflammation found on their final histopathologic examination [11]. The purpose of this study was to evaluate the predictive value of the severity assessment classification of cholecystitis using the Tokyo Guidelines, as well as follow outcomes of each severity grade. In general, the authors found a statistically significant correlation between increasing preoperative severity grade and the extent of gallbladder inflammation on final histopathology. However, they also found that over 40% of patients with grade I acute cholecystitis had pathology consistent with advanced cholecystitis. This suggests that the Tokyo Guidelines may downgrade the degree of inflammation at the time of presentation. When following outcomes, patients with grade II/III cholecystitis were significantly more likely to have postoperative complications as well as a conversion from laparoscopic to open procedure [11]. It is important to keep in mind the limitations of this study. First, it should be noted that both Grades II and III, per the Tokyo Guidelines, can be managed with percutaneous cholecysostomy tube and thus no final histopathologic examination can be performed. This fact limited the power of these two groups, and thus Grades II and III were lumped into a single group. Additionally, the Guidelines recommendation for Grade III is generally *not* surgical intervention, further limiting this cohort. While it is not surprising that Grades II/III have higher operative complications and conversions to open when compared to Grade I, further studies are needed to compare the outcomes of severity Grade II vs Grade III.

Wright and colleagues also examined patient outcomes using the Tokyo Guidelines (TG) for diagnosis and severity. They performed a single institution, retrospective review of all patients who presented with acute cholecystitis over a 5 year period, creating three cohorts based on TG severity assessment (Group 1 = Grade I, Group 2 = Grade II, Group 3 = Grade III). They found significantly increased length of stay, disposition to home, and morbidity based on increasing severity of disease [2]. For the patients who underwent operative intervention, higher severity grade was associated with increased conversion to an open procedure, increased operative time, increased length of stay, disposition to home, and increased readmission [2]. Compared to studies conducted in Asia, this study, which was performed in the United States, had a higher percentage of males and obese patients. Furthermore, this study had more patients present with Grade II severity. This was in opposition to the Asian studies, which had a high percentage of patient's presenting with Grade I severity. In this study, patients met Grade II severity criteria primarily due to the fact that they presented with symptoms for more than 72 hours. The authors hypothesized that patients in the United States could have a more indolent disease course, or that they are less likely to urgently seek medical attention [2]. The authors also stress that the results of the study provide a framework of anticipated outcomes based on severity grading. They feel this is vitally important as the United States moves toward a pay for performance model of reimbursement.

Several other studies have shown similar correlations between Tokyo severity grade and length of stay and complications. In a retrospective review, Cheng et al. showed a statistically significant increase in length of stay and complication rate based on increasing TG severity grade of acute cholecystitis [13]. A similar correlation was seen between length of stay and Charlson's Comorbidity Scores [13]. In an interesting side note, this study found that patient management was not always congruent with that recommended by the Tokyo Guidelines. Given this was a retrospective study, this is not surprising. Specifically, the Guidelines describe treatment for Grade I disease as monitored medical therapy or early operative intervention. In this study, 48 patients presented with Grade I acute cholecystitis. While 17 were treated with antibiotics and 18 were treated with cholecystectomy, 13 were treated with cholecystostomy tube [13]. This incongruence was believed to be due to the surgeon's evaluation of the patients' comorbidities in determining the best treatment modality. In another retrospective review of patients presenting with acute cholecystitis, Ni et al. also used the Tokyo Guidelines to grade the severity of the disease at presentation [12]. They were then able to isolate those who were eligible for surgery or percutaneous transhepatic gallbladder drainage. They found that patients who were elderly and those with comorbidities were better candidates for percutaneous drainage with the purpose of quickly alleviating symptoms [12].

MANAGEMENT OF GRADE II (MODERATE) ACUTE CHOLECYSTITIS

The Tokyo Guidelines define Grade II or moderate acute cholecystitis as cholecystitis associated with one of the following clinical findings : 1) Elevated WBC (>18000), 2) Palpable tender mass in the right upper quadrant, 3) Duration of complaints more than 72 hours, or 4) Marked local inflammation (biliary peritonitis, pericholecystic abscess, hepatic abscess, gangrenous or emphysematous cholecystitis) [8]. With this definition, a patient can present with one of these findings, two of these findings, three of these findings, or even all four. In all of these scenarios, the patient has the same severity grading. This illustrates the wide variety of clinical presentation in those with Grade II disease. The authors feel that a patient with one of these findings versus a patient with all four findings represent different clinical entities. This creates controversy in selecting the appropriate treatment modality as Grade II patients likely cover a broader clinical spectrum than that of a single severity grade. Further complicating the matter, the Tokyo Guidelines do not account for age or comorbid conditions, both of which further extend the breadth of disease severity in patients described with Grade II disease. With such a wide spectrum of clinical presentations in a single severity classification, it is not surprising that the most recent Guidelines reflect this and suggest an algorithm in their management recommendations:

> "Grade II (moderate) acute cholecystitis is often accompanied by severe local inflammation. Therefore, surgeons should take the difficulty of cholecystectomy into consideration in selecting a treatment method Elective cholecystectoy after the improvement of the acute inflammatory process is the first-line treatment. If a patient does not respond to initial medical treatment, urgent or early gallbladder drainage is required. Early laparoscopic cholecystectomy could be indicated if advanced laparoscopic techniques are available. Grade II (moderate)

acute cholecystitis with serious local complications is an indication for urgent cholecystectomy and drainage."

The dilemma lies in the following question: which Grade II patients are best managed with medical therapy and drainage versus those best managed with cholecystectomy? Furthermore, what is the ideal timing of an operation if indicated?

Drainage Procedures

Cholecystostomy tube placement can be performed operatively or percutaneously with radiology guidance. Currently, it is commonly used to temporize patients with acute cholecystitis who are not operative candidates due to comorbidities, age, severe infection, shock or in those without access to surgical treatment. The efficacy of cholecystostomy tubes resolving acute cholecystitis is 61-100% [14]. Complications such as biliary leak, biliary peritonitis, biliary fistula, and bleeding range from 0-12.5% [14]. Mortality for the procedure is 0-38% [14]. It is proposed that older patients with significant comorbidities and advanced cholecystitis benefit most from cholecystostomy tube placement. However, their use remains institution dependent, with no accepted guidelines for identifying patients who benefit from the procedure.

The Tokyo Guidelines do not take into account the age or comorbidities of a patient in assigning them to a severity classification or recommending treatment. Historically, patients who present with acute cholecystitis who are older or have more comorbidities were more likely to undergo cholecystostomy tube placement instead of cholecystectomy. Cull et al. performed a retrospective study reviewing the management of over 800 patients over the age of 65 years old who presented with biliary complaints [15]. Patients were sorted into one of three groups based on whether they underwent 1) cholecystostomy tube placement then interval cholecystectomy, 2) early cholecystectomy, or 3) delayed cholecystectomy [15]. Despite the belief that cholecystostomy tube placement may decrease risks associated with cholecystectomy, they showed that there was no difference between the groups in regard to conversion to open, biliary leak, bowel injury, and reoperation. Furthermore, they showed that those who had a percutaneous cholecystostomy tube placed followed by interval cholecystectomy were more likely to have recurrent cholecystitis, pancreatitis, and cholangitis in comparison to those who had early cholecystectomy. This suggests that advanced age alone should not be the determining factor used to identify patients who would best benefit from cholecystostomy tube placement.

Even in patients with significant comorbidities, operative cholecystectomy is generally preferred over percutaneous cholecystostomy at institutions that have a high operative volume and surgeons who are skilled in laparoscopy. Kamalapurkar et al. showed successful management of moderate and severe cholecystitis with operative intervention [16]. Of 84 patients who presented with moderate or severe acute cholecystitis, 88% underwent cholecystectomy with only 3 of the patients with severe cholecystitis having undergone cholecystostomy tube placement [16]. Overall, conversion to an open procedure and length of stay were increased in those with Grade III disease. However, there was no significant increase in morbidity in the cohort who had cholecystectomy compared to those treated non operatively. This may suggest that patients with grade II disease may be best treated with initial operative cholecystectomy.

Operative Intervention and Strategies

Although there are situations in which the use of percutaneous cholecystostomy tube is appropriate, cholecystectomy remains the gold standard for the treatment of acute cholecystitis in the appropriate clinical context. Patients with Grade II (moderate) acute cholecystitis are the most varied in presentation, as well as operative findings. Thus the surgeon needs to be prepared for a wide variety of intraoperative scenarios. Laparoscopic cholecystectomy has become the mainstay in the operative management of cholecystitis and should remain in the forefront even in those with Grade II disease. Numerous strategies have been established to complete this operation in a safe and reproducible manner, even in cases with difficult and acutely inflamed gallbladders, i.e., those seen in Grade II cholecystitis. One such strategy is establishing the Critical View of Safety (CVoS). In this method, the surgeon must meet three criteria prior to clipping and transecting the ductal structures. First, two and only two structures must be noted entering the infundibulum of the gallbladder. Second, the lower third of the gallbladder must be dissected off the liver (i.e., gallbladder fossa), revealing the cystic plate. Finally, all fibro-fatty tissue between the cystic duct and artery must be cleared. Another strategy is the use of intraoperative imaging to help confirm or identify pertinent anatomy and structures. These include intraoperative cholangiogram and ultrasound.

Situations do exist in which, despite the use of intraoperative imaging such as ultrasound and cholangiogram, the critical view of safety cannot be established laparoscopically. In these situations it has historically been recommended that the operation be converted to open. In today's age of laparoscopy, this is often viewed as a failure. Some studies propose that converting to an open procedure during cholecystectomy leads to longer duration of stay and increased post-operative complications. Therefore, Asai et al. performed a retrospective study to identify patient characteristics that increase their chance to have a procedure convert to open [17]. A univariate analysis identified these characteristics as duration of symptoms greater than 72 hours, elevated CRP, and increased Tokyo Guidelines severity grade [17].

While conversion to open in difficult laparoscopic cases is certainly a valid option, bailout procedures are well established and are becoming more accepted and common in the management of technically challenging laparoscopic cholecystectomies. Partial gallbladder removal in the open operation was first described in 1898 by Hans Kehr, during which he left the posterior wall and infundibulum due to difficult conditions [18]. Since that time, variations of partial cholecystectomy have been developed. These bailout procedures include subtotal cholecystectomy: fenestrated or reconstituting. A recent article in the Journal of the American College of Surgeons by leading experts in the field of biliary surgery describes these procedures in depth. For subtotal fenestrating cholecystectomy, the posterior wall of the gallbladder and a lip of the lowest portion of the peritonealized portion of the gallbladder are left in place [19]. The gallstones are then extracted and the mucosa is ablated. While the cut edge may be oversewn or the cystic duct can be closed from the inside with a purse string suture, the gallbladder itself is left open. This bypasses the need to ligate the cystic duct, which in the setting of significant inflammation, can lead to common bile duct injury [19]. For subtotal reconstituting cholecystectomy, the posterior gallbladder wall can be completely or partially left in situ while the entirety of the peritonealized gallbladder is removed [19]. The reconstitution results in an intact lumen in which stones can reform and symptoms can return [19]. These additional surgical strategies help avoid intraoperative morbidity and allow for successful completion of a safe and effective operation. Despite the fact that laparoscopic cholecystectomy is the preferred operative treatment for acute cholecystitis, it is important to recognize that conversion to an open procedure should not be considered a failure as long as the procedure is completed safely [1].

Timing of Operation

While ideal first line management of patients with Grade II (moderate) acute cholecystitis is cholecystectomy, the timing of operative intervention is controversial. Many proceed with caution to the OR, as patients who present with acute cholecystitis can have a significant inflammatory response that can distort anatomy and increase the difficulty of completing the procedure safely. In a report by the Cochrane Database of Systematic Reviews, a higher number of patients with common bile duct injuries were seen in those who underwent early cholecystectomy compared to delayed cholecystectomy [20]. However, other studies have shown early cholecystectomy to decrease length of stay *without* increasing morbidity [21]. In theory, patients with mild (Grade I) acute cholecystitis do not have as much inflammation as those with more severe disease (Grades II and III). This should make operative intervention less technically challenging, making the decision for early operation easier for surgeons and patients in Grade I disease. Furthermore, the degree of inflammation, and thus severity of cholecystitis, progresses with time. Thus, it would seem advantageous to pursue early intervention when possible. This is evident by the fact that in the Tokyo Guidelines, one of the criteria that advances a patient from Grade I (mild) disease to Grade II (moderate) disease, is the presence of symptoms for *greater* than 72 hours.

Several studies have been conducted to assess the advantage of early versus delayed cholecystectomy, with the definition of early being variable (from within 72 hours of presentation to within 7 days of presentation). Menahem et al. performed a meta analysis of randomized controlled trials looking at this topic [21]. Nine prospective randomized trials were included. They compared the 617 patients who underwent early laparoscopic cholecystectomy (ELC) to 603 patients who underwent delayed laparoscopic cholecystectomy (DLC) for acute cholecystitis (32). The mean hospital stay was statistically significantly lower in the ELC compared to the DLC (5.4 days versus 9.1 days, respectively) [21]. Additionally, the incidence of major biliary duct injury was equivocal (0.8% versus 0.9%). The definition of early versus delayed laparoscopic cholecystectomy varied based on individual study, with most including patients who underwent an operation within 72 hours of presentation [21]. Polo et al. also examined the timing of cholecystectomy by reviewing the French national health care database. They selected all patients who underwent cholecystectomy over a three year period, which included 42,452 patients from 507 hospitals. Those who had surgery within 3 days of admission had significantly less post operative complications such as ICU admission, reoperation, and sepsis (3-3.3%, 0.5-0.6%, and 3.8-4.1%) compared to those who had surgery beyond the first 3 admission days (4.5%, 1%, and 6.5%) [22]. These studies suggest that early laparoscopic cholecystectomy is advantageous to delayed laparoscopic cholecystectomy.

While many agree that early cholecystectomy is preferred (certainly within 72 hours), debate still exists with regards to the extent of an "early cholecystectomy." Essentially, at what time period does "early" transition to "delayed." Is it within 96 hours, as suggested by the TG13 mobile application, where, under severity assessment, Grade II has the recommendation of "cholecystectomy within 96 hours of symptoms?" This distinction may seem minute, but when looking at the inclusion criteria for Grade II (moderate) acute cholecystitis, one criterion is the presence of symptoms greater than 72 hours. This criterion, while placing a patient in Grade II, also places them out of the "window" for early cholecystectomy by many study and practical definitions.

CONCLUSION

Overall, the Tokyo Guidelines provide an excellent framework for the diagnosis, grading, and management of acute cholecystitis. Numerous institutions around the world have implemented these Guidelines into practice. Studies have been published, with retrospective data demonstrating correlation between severity grade and histopathologic examination. Additionally, studies show that with increasing severity grade, the length of stay, conversion to open, and complication rate all increase. Despite the acceptance of the diagnostic and severity grading parameters described in the Guidelines, there remains significant variability in the management of acute cholecystitis. This is explained by the varying degrees of biliary inflammation. The Guidelines looked to stratify these degrees of inflammation by creating the severity assessment or grades of acute cholecystitis. This allowed for a more specific treatment algorithm for each grade. While the management of Grade I (mild) and Grade III (severe) are generally straightforward, Grade II disease represents a wider spectrum of the clinical presentation of acute cholecystitis. While some institutions advocate uniformity in management (specifically, that all patients should undergo cholecystectomy at the time of presentation), others propose the use of additional parameters beyond those described in the Tokyo Guidelines, such as age and comorbidities, to identify patients who would benefit from medical therapy versus cholecystostomy versus cholecystectomy.

Based on the available literature, the authors feel that patients presenting with Grade II (moderate) acute cholecystitis should undergo laparoscopic cholecystectomy if at all possible. This is contingent on the surgeon being comfortable with advanced laparoscopy and the patient being an appropriate operative candidate (i.e., taking into account comorbidities). We do not feel advanced age alone is enough to keep the patient out of the operating room if they are a suitable candidate. If a patient is determined to be unfit for the operating room, then medical therapy and percutaneous cholecystostomy are appropriate alternatives. If the operation is technically challenging and the critical view of safety (CVoS) is unable to be obtained, intraoperative imaging should be attempted in the form of cholangiogram or ultrasound. If the CVoS is still unable to be obtained, then the surgeon has the option to 1) convert to open, 2) perform a laparoscopic bailout procedure (subtotal fenestrating cholecystectomy versus subtotal reconstituting cholecystectomy), or 3) terminate the procedure after operative cholecystostomy tube placement. We favor a laparoscopic bailout procedure. With regards to the timing of the operation, the authors advocate early cholecystectomy (within 72 hours) when possible. In those situations when patients present outside of this time window (i.e., past 72 hours), urgent percutaneous cholecystostomy tube placement, urgent cholecystectomy, and medical management (the so called "cool off period") followed by delayed cholecystectomy are all reasonable. Further studies are needed to identify which of these management strategies will most benefit patients in this small sub classification of Grade II (moderate) acute cholecystitis.

REFERENCES

[1] Kimura, Y., Takada, T., Strasberg, S. M., Pitt, H. A., Gouma, D. J., Garden, O. J., Buchler, M. W., Windsor, J. A., Mayumi, T., Yoshida, M., Miura, F., Higuchi, R., Gabata, T., Hata, J., Gomi, H., Dervenis, C., Lau, W. Y., Gelli, G., Kim, M. H., Hilvano, S. C. and Yamashita, Y. (2013). TG13 current terminology, etiology, and epidemiology of acute cholangitis and cholecystitis. *J Hepatobiliary Pancreat Sci.*, *20*, 8-23.

[2] Wright, G. P., Stilwell, K., Johnson, J., Hefty, M. T. and Chung M. H. (2015). Predicting length of stay and conversion to open cholecystectomy for acute cholecystitis using the 2013 Tokyo

Guidelines in a US population. *J Hepatobiliary Pancreat Sci., 22*, 795-801.

[3] Sekimoto, M., Takada, T., Kawarada, Y., Nimura, Y., Yoshida, M., Mayumi, T., Miura, F., Wada, K., Hirota, M., Yamashita, Y., Strasberg, S., Pitt, H. A., Belghiti, J., Santibanes, E., Gadacz, T. R., Hilvano, S. C., Kim, S. Q., Liau, K. H., Fan, S. T., Belli, G. and Sachakul, V. (2007). Need for criteria for the diagnosis and severity assessment of acute cholangitis and cholecystitis: Tokyo Guidelines. *J Hepatobiliary Pancreat Sci., 14*, 11-14.

[4] Kim, W. R., Brown, R. S., Terrault, N. A. and El-Serag, H. (2002). Burden of liver disease in the United States summary of a workshop. *Hepatology., 36*, 227-242.

[5] Yokoe, M., Takada, T., Mayumi, T., Yoshida, M., Hasegawa, H., Norimizu, S., Hayashi, K., Umemura, S. and Orito, E. (2011). Accuracy of the Tokyo Guidelines for the diagnosis of acute cholangitis and cholecystitis taking into consideration the clinical practice pattern in Japan. *J Hepatobiliary Pacreat Sci., 18*, 250-257.

[6] Strasberg, S. M. (2008). Acute calculous cholecystitis. *N Engl J Med., 358*, 2804-2811.

[7] Takada, T., Kawarada, Y., Nimura, Y., Yoshida, M., Maumi, T., Sekimoto, M., Miura, F., Wada, K., Hirota, M., Yamashita, Y., Nagino, M., Tsuyuguchi, T., Tanaka, A., Kimura, Y., Yasuda, H., Hirata, K., Pitt, H. A., Strasberge, S. m., Gadacz, T. F., Bornman, P. C., Gouma, D. J., Belli, G. and Liau, K. H. (2007). Background: Tokyo Guidelines for the management of acute cholangitis and cholecystitis. *J Hepatobiliary Pacreat Sci., 14*, 1-10.

[8] Mayumi, T., Takada, T., Kawarada, Y., Nimura, Y., Yoshida, M., Sekimoto, M., Miura, F., Wada, K., Hirota, M., Yamashita, Y., Nagino, M., Tsuyuguchi, T., Tanaka, A., Gomi, H. and Pitt, H. A. (2007). Results of the Tokyo Consensus Meeting Tokyo Guidelines. *J Hepatobiliary Pancreat Surg., 14*, 114-121.

[9] Takada, T., Strasberg, S. M., Solomkin, J. S., Pitt, H. A., Gomi, H., Yoshida, M., Mayumi, T., Miura, F., Gouma, D. J., Garden, O. J., Buchler, M. W., Kiriyama, S., Yokoe, M., Kimura, Y., Tsuyuguchi, T., Itoi, T., Gabata, T., Higuchi, R., Okamoto, K., Hata, J., Murata, A., Kusachi, S., Windsor, J. A., Supe, A. N., Lee, S. G., Chen, X. P., Yamashita, Y., Hirata, K., Inui, K. and Sumiyama, Y. (2013). TG13: Updated Tokyo Guidelines for the management of acute cholangitis and cholecystitis. *J Hepatobiliary Pancreat Sci., 20*, 1-7.

[10] Lee, S. W., Yang, S. S., Chang, C. S. and Yeh, H. J. (2009). Impact of the Tokyo guidelines on the management of patients with acute calculous cholecystitis. *J Gastroen Hepatol.*, *24*, 1857-1861.

[11] Ambe, P. C., Christ, H. and Wassenberg, D. (2015). Does the Tokyo Guidelines predict the extent of gallbladder inflammation in patients with acute cholecystitis? A single center retrospective analysis. *BMC Gastroenterology.*, *15*, 142-149.

[12] Ni, Q., Chen, D., Xu, R. and Shang, D. (2015). The Efficacy of Percutaneous Transhepatic Gallbladder Drainage on Acute Cholecystitis in High-Risk Elderly Patients Based on the Tokyo Guidelines. *Medicine.*, *94*(34), 1442-1448.

[13] Cheng, W. C., Chiu, Y. C., Chuang, C. H. and Chen, C. Y. (2014). Assessing clinical outcomes of patients with acute calculous cholecystitis in addition to the Tokyo grading: A retrospective study. *Kaohsiung J Med Sci.*, *30*, 459-465.

[14] Rodriguez-Sanjuan, J. C., Arruabarrena, A., Sanchez-Moreno, L., Gonzalez-Sanchez, F., Herrera, L. A. and Gomez-Fleitas, M. (2012). Acute cholecystitis in high surgical risk patients, percutaneous cholecystostomy or emergency cholecystectomy. *Am J Surg.*, *204*(1), 54-59.

[15] Cull, J. D., Velasco, J. M., Czubak, A., Rice, D. and Brown, E. C. (2013). Management of Acute Cholecystitis: Prevalence of Percutaneous Cholecystostomy and Delayed Cholecystectomy in the Elderly. *J Gastrointest Surg.*, *18*, 328-333.

[16] Kamalapurkar, D., Pang, T. C. Y., Siriwardhane, M., Hollands, M., Johnston, E., Pleass, H., Richardson, A. and Lam, V. W. (2015). Index cholecystectomy in grade II and II acute calculous cholecystitis is feasible and safe. *Anz J Surg.*, *85*, 854-859.

[17] Asai, K., Watanabe, M., Kusachi, S., Matsukiyo, H., Saito, T., Kodama, H., Kiribayashi, T., Enomoto, T., Nakamura, Y., Okamoto, Y., Saida, Y. and Nagao, J. (2014). Risk factors for conversion of laparoscopic cholecystectomy to open surgery associated with the severity characteristics according to the Tokyo guidelines. *Surg Today.*, *44*, 2300-2304.

[18] Kehr, H. (1901). Introduction to the Differential Diagnosis of the Separate Forms of Gallstone Disease: Based upon His Own Experience Gained from 433 Laparotomies for Gallstones. Philadelphia: P Blakiston's Son and Co.

[19] Strasberg, S. M., Pucci, M. J., Brunt, M. and Deziel, D. J. (2016). Subtotal Cholecystectomy—"Fenestrating" vs "Reconstituting" Subtypes and the Prevention of Bile Duct Injury: Definition of the Optimal Procedure in Difficult Operative Conditions. *J Am Coll Surg.*, *222*(1), 89-96.

[20] Gurusamy, K. S. and Samraj, K. (2006). Early versus delayed laparoscopic cholecystectomy for acute cholecystitis. *Cochrane Database Syst Rev.*, *4*, CD005440.

[21] Menahem, B., Mulliri, A., Fohlen, A., Guittet, L., Alves, A. and Lubrano, J. (2015). Delayed laparoscopic cholecystectomy increases the total hospital stay compared to an early laparoscopic cholecystectomy after acute cholecystitis: an updated meta-analysis of randomized controlled trials. *HPB.*, 17, 857-862.

[22] Polo, M., Duclos, A., Polazzi, S., Payet, C., Lifante, J. C., Cotte, E., Barth, X., Glehen, O. and Passot, G. (2015). Acute Cholecystitis—Optimal Timing for Early Cholecystectomy: a French Nationwide Study. *J Gastrointest Surg.*, *19*(11), 2003-2010.

[23] Asai, K., Watanabe, M., Kusachi, S., Tanaka, H., Matsukiyo, H., Osawa, A., Saito, T., Kodama, H., Enomoto, T., Nakamura, Y., Okamoto, Y., Saida, Y. and Nagao, J. (2012). Bacteriological analysis of bile in acute cholecystitis according to the Tokyo guidelines. *J Hepatobiliary Pancreat Sci.*, *19*, 476-486.

[24] Fujii, Y., Ohuchida, J., Chijiiwa, K., Yano, K., Imamura, N., Nagano, M., Hiyoshi, M., Otani, K., Kai, M. and Kondo, K. (2012). Verification of Tokyo Guidelines for diagnosis and management of acute cholangitis. *J Hepatobiliary Pancreat Sci.*, *19*, 487-491.

[25] Yokoe, M., Takada, T., Strasberg, S. M., Solomkin, J. S., Mayumi, T., Gomi, H., Pitt, H. A., Garden, O. J., Kiriyama, S., Hata, J., Gabata, T., Yoshida, M., Miura, F., Okamoto, K., Tsuyuguchi, T., Itoi, T., Yamashita, Y., Dervenis, C., Chan, A. C. W., Lau, W. Y., Supe, A. N., Belli, G., Hilvano, S. C., Liau, K. H., Kim, M. H., Kim, S. W. and Ker, C. G. (2013). *TG13 diagnostic criteria and severity grading of acute cholecystitis.*, 20, 35-46.

[26] Tsuyuguchi, T., Itoi, T., Takada, T., Strasberg, S. M., Pitt, H. A., Kim, M. H., Supe, A. N., Mayumi, T., Yoshida, M., Miura, F., Gomi, H., Kimura, Y., Higuchi, R., Okamoto, K., Tamashita, Y., Gabata, T., Hata, J. and Kusachi, S. (2013). TG13 indications and techniques for gallbladder drainage in acute cholecystitis. *J Hepatobiliary Pancreat Sci.*, *20*, 81-88.

In: Acute Cholecystitis
Editor: Lisa Powell

ISBN: 978-1-63485-744-4

Chapter 6

CHOLECYSTITIS IN SYSTEMIC LUPUS ERYTHEMATOSUS

Thouraya Ben Salem* and Imed Ben Ghorbel

Department of Internal Medicine, La Rabta University Hopital Tunis, Tunisia

Faculty of Medicine, University El Manar, Tunis, Tunisia

ABSTRACT

Gastrointestinal (GI) manifestations of systemic lupus erythematosus (SLE) are common. Any part of the GI tract can be involved but cholecystitis is rare in SLE patients. Only a few cases are reported. Cholecystitis can be an initial manifestation of SLE or can occur in the disease course, in association with other severe involvements. Clinical presentation is non-specific. Patients have abdominal pain, vomiting and fever. Examination can reveal right upper quadrant tenderness. Symptoms can be attenuated by the use of corticosteroid when patients are already treated for SLE. Laboratory data can show increased level of liver enzymes. Ultrasonography may show gallbladder thickness wall with or without pericholecystic edema and in most of cases, there are no signs of lithiasis. Abdominal computed tomography confirms the diagnosis showing gallbladder wall thickness and edema.

When cholecystectomy is performed, histological examination confirms the inflammation and in most cases shows vasculitis which can

* E-mail: bensalemthouraya@yahoo.fr.

be associated with fibrinoid necrosis. Otherwise, thromboembolic events with or without antiphospholipid antibodies can be responsible for acute cholecystitis.

In the absence of controlled trials, treatment of acalculous cholecystitis is based on clinical experiences. High dose steroid may be the first line therapy but other immunosuppressant agents (cyclophosphamide, azathiorpine) can be considered. Anticoagulants are used when thrombosis is identified as a cause. Cholecystectomy is often performed in patients when cholecystitis inaugurates the disease and SLE is not yet diagnosed. In other cases, patients may undergo surgery when medical treatment is ineffective.

Keywords: systemic lupus erythematosus, cholecystitis, abdominal pain, vasculitis

INTRODUCTION

Systemic lupus erythematosus (SLE) is an autoimmune disease characterized by a wide spectrum of clinical manifestations and the presence of multiple autoantibodies. The most frequent manifestations of this chronic inflammatory disease are cutaneous and articular involvements and the most serious are renal and cardiac complications. Gastrointestinal (GI) manifestations in SLE are common. Their prevalence is variable and depends on whether investigations are performed routinely or not. Prevalence varies widely from 1.3 to 27.5% [18]. Abdominal pain is frequent in SLE, reported in 5.5 to 40% of patients [18, 21] and can be directly related to SLE, caused by medications or due to non-SLE etiologies. Abdominal pain is the major symptom revealing GI involvements in SLE patients. Among them, mesenteric vasculitis and pancreatitis are the most frequent. Other causes including appendicitis, acute gastroenteritis, and peritonitis may be considered [21]. Acalculous cholecystitis (AC) is uncommon in SLE patients and only a few cases were reported.

Prevalence

AC is a rare abdominal manifestation in SLE; its prevalence is probably under-estimated since it is not systematically screened like serious and frequent manifestations of lupus (renal, central neurological or cardiac complications). There are no real data for this prevalence. In all SLE series, AC is discussed as a cause of abdominal pain and rarely listed as a single manifestation of SLE. It seems that AC is the less frequent cause of abdominal pain in SLE patients. In a study of 126 SLE patients who were hospitalized because of acute abdominal pain, 6.2% had cholecystitis whereas pancreatitis was noted in 10.3% of them [20]. In a series of 201 children with SLE, 39 presented with abdominal pain (19%), and among them one had AC (0.4%) [15]. In our experience, among 266 SLE patients, four had AC (1.5%). In one case, AC revealed the SLE [5]. Case reports of AC revealing or complicating the SLE course were reported [7, 8, 14]. Furthermore, in a study of 67 children with acalculous diffuse gallbladder wall thickening, only two patients had SLE [11].

Circumstance of Discovery and Clinical Features

Clinical presentation of AC is non-specific and in most cases, patients complain of abdominal pain in the right upper quadrant. Nausea, vomiting and fever are frequently associated to abdominal pain, mimicking acute surgery abdomen. Symptoms may also be neglected and attributed to medications such as non steroids anti-inflammatory drugs, hydroxychloroquine or azathiorpine.

In many patients who are already treated with corticosteroids and immunosuppressive drugs, symptoms can be mild or absent. AC can be completely asymptomatic and discovered by abdominal ultrasound or revealed by liver enzymes increase.

At examination, tenderness in the right upper quadrant with positive Murphy's sign is noted. Abdomen examination can be unremarkable.

Biological Data

All liver enzymes: aspartate amino transferase (AST), alanine amino transferase, alkaline phosphatase, glutamyl transpeptidase (GGT) and bilirubin can rise in patients with AC.

A biological inflammatory syndrome may also be noted but procalcitonin is negative.

Biological findings may show hematological abnormalities (anemia, leucopenia and thrombocytopenia) as signs of SLE relapse. Positive proteinuria and renal failure may be noted and are signs of lupus nephritis flare. Antinuclear and anti-DNA antibodies are positive in most cases and complement fractions (C3, C4 and CH50) are decreased, showing that the disease is active.

Exceptionally, patients with AC may not present any biological abnormalities [17].

Imaging

AC is confirmed using sonography. Abdominal ultrasound shows gallbladder wall thickening with or without pericholecystic edema. Gallbladder can be distended without signs stones. Abdominal ultrasound may also reveal associated complications in SLE patients like peritonitis and ascites [17] and screen other manifestations such as hepatomegaly and splenomegaly [12]. Abdominal computed tomography is indicated for better assessment, when ultrasound is not contributive or inconclusive. Computed tomography shows gallbladder wall thickening and edema confirming sonography abnormalities. Abdominal scan is needed to rule out other abdominal pain causes such as pancreatitis.

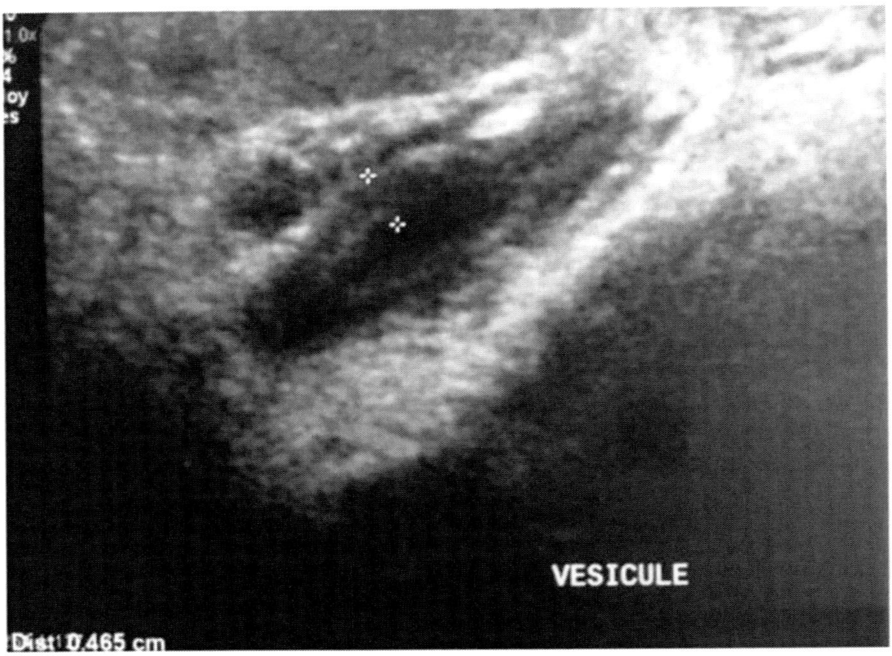

Abdominal untrasound: Gallbladder wall thickening in a woman with systemic lupus erythematosus.

Diagnosis

Abdominal pain in patient with a history of SLE, biochemical abnormalities and typical abdominal sonography findings can lead to AC diagnosis. In most series, AC occurs in active SLE, and is often associated with other severe lupus manifestations especially lupus nephritis and cardiac complications [3-5]. In such patients, AC isn't the first interest of physicians who are naturally focused in serious complications. AC diagnosis is suspected when abdominal pain persists despite treatment (corticosteroids with or without immunosuppressive therapy). Other abdominal pain etiologies like appendicitis, pancreatitis, intestinal vasculitis or mesenteric and other abdominal veins thromboses can be seen in SLE patients and must be ruled out. Many of them may occur in the same patient at the same time or may be associated with AC [3].

AC happens in patients with a new disease relapse with a delay to SLE diagnosis of some years [2, 7]. Among our patients, two had AC during SLE relapses with a mean delay of 7 years was associated with myo-pericarditis in one case and with pulmonary hypertension in other patient. AC symptoms may appear a few days or weeks after starting treatment of a new lupus relapse [19]. In these cases, digestive perforation is firstly suspected because patients are given high dose steroids and AC diagnosis is delayed.

Exceptionally, AC occurred in a patient with SLE history without any other signs or symptoms of the disease [17].

In patients with long history of SLE, who are receiving low dose of steroids, lack of abdominal pain at the moment of AC may be a cause of diagnosis delay.

Otherwise, AC occurs during the first SLE flare, when the disease is not already known. A few cases of AC revealing SLE were reported [5, 12]. Diagnosis is established since AC is commonly concomitant to other SLE involvements [5, 8, 14] with positive antinuclear antibodies and low complement fractions.

SLE related AC is more difficult to diagnosis in the absence of other lupus symptoms which may be delayed and appear on the disease course [8].

Acute AC may also complicate drug induced lupus. This was reported in one case and cholecystitis was associated with polyserositis [16].

In the absence of signs of lupus flare, abdominal pain is most likely due to conventional surgical disorders. Sometimes it isn't easy to distinguish SLE related AC from infectious cholecystitis. Infections are a frequent complication in SLE patients and should be screened. In all patients, other causes of gallbladder wall thickening should be ruled out: infections, acute hepatitis or pancreatitis and specific liver disease [11].

Calculous cholecystitis may be seen in SLE patients. Microlithiasis is not uncommon in SLE patients especially those with chronic hemolysis. Hemolysis is consistently associated with a higher risk of developing gallstones. But presence of microlithiases doesn't exclude SLE related AC since both conditions can be associated [2, 9].

Histopathology

Histopathological findings are obtained when surgery is conducted. Vasculitis is the most frequent abnormality found in SLE patients with AC [19, 20]. Necrotizing vasculitis involves small and medium vessels [2, 4] and can be associated with mesenteric vasculitis [2]. Acute inflammation may be noted but signs of chronic cholecystitis are also reported [2, 20]. In addition, thrombosis and ischemic lesion are described in patients with or without antiphospholipid syndrome [9, 19].

In patients with gallstones, presence of vasculitis in histological examination confirms that both conditions co-exist [2, 9].

Treatment

Corticosteroids

In patients with SLE history and with other organ involvements, AC is easily related to SLE and conservative treatment should be considered. High dose oral corticosteroids with or without methylprednisone pulses are sufficient and efficient [5, 10, 12]. But in most cases, immunosuppressive drugs are added to treat severe manifestations like lupus nephritis, neurological or cardiac involvements [8, 14].

Some patients have antibiotics initially until infectious causes are ruled out [8, 12]. In the absence of infection, corticosteroids are added.

Cholecystectomy

In a few cases, absence of improvement despite corticosteroids and immunopressive therapy lead to cholecystectomy [4], especially when infection is still suspected [6].

Surgery is performed in emergency when SLE diagnosis is not already established [15] because calculous cholecystitis and infection are still the first suspected diagnoses. Contrasting with the ancient reports [1], in recent cases, surgery is less performed. We think that now days, SLE related AC is well known even in surgical units and when patients presented initially with AC, they are conferred to rheumatologist. Otherwise, cholecystectomy is performed in patients with gallstones [2, 9] since before histological examination it is impossible to distinguish gallstones complication from SLE related inflammation of the gallbladder. When signs of AC follow other lupus symptoms and steroids are already started, patients may undergo surgery [19] because of suspected digestive perforation.

Outcome

Complete remission of AC is usual, abdominal pain is healed after medical treatment or after surgery. If cholecystectomy is not performed, abdominal ultrasound shows that signs of AC disappear.

Mortality in patients with AC is probably related to other associated lupus serious manifestations or cardiac complications [2].

In a study evaluating abdominal pain in SLE patients, the death rate was 38.8% in patients with active SLE and was 13.3% in cases of inactive disease [13].

REFERENCES

[1] Al Hakeem MS, Mc Millen MA. Evaluation of abdominal pain in systemic lupus erythematosus. *Am. J. Surg.,* 1998, 176, 291-4.

[2] Ashouri JF, Davis JL, Farkas A, Durack JC, Ramachandran R, Dall'Era M. A young woman with systemic lupus erythematosus and extensive mesenteric vasculitis involving small and medium vessels. *Arthritis Care Res.* (Hoboken), 2012 Dec, 64(12), 1928-33.

[3] Barrera-Ramirez CF, Pineda-Pompa LR, Melo M, Valdez Castro R, Medina-Gomez H, Godina-Alonso G, Guzman CE. Hemorrhagic pericarditis and cardiac tamponade in systemic lupus erythematosus. A case report. *Arch. Cardiol. Mex.*, 2005 Jul-Sep, 75 Suppl 3, S3-96-9.

[4] Basiratnia M, Vasei M, Bahador A, Ebrahimi E, Derakhshan A. Acute acalculous cholecystitis in a child with systemic lupus erythematosus. *Pediatr. nephrol.*, 2006 Jun, 21(6), 873-6.

[5] Ben Ghorbel I, Souabni L, Lamloum M, Khanfir M, Braham A, Miled M, Houman H. Systemic lupus erythematosus revealed by acute acalculous cholecystitis. *Gastroenterol. Clin. Biol.*, 2009 Dec, 33(12), 1175-6.

[6] Blaauw AA, Tobé TJ, Derksen RW, Bijlsma JW. A patient with systemic lupus erythematosus and salmonella enteritidis bacteraemia complicated by rhabdomyolysis and acute cholecystitis. *Rheumatology* (Oxford), 2000, 39, 110-2.

[7] Cheng YL, Lee KC, Luo JC. A young woman presenting with jaundice. *Gastroenterology*, 2012, 143(2), e1-2.

[8] Choi YJ, Yoon HY, Jang SA, Hong MJ, Lee WS, Yoo WH. A case of systemic lupus erythematosus initially presented with acute acalculous cholecystitis. *J. Rheum. Dis.*, 2014, 21, 140-2.

[9] De-Leon-Bojorge B, Zaltzman-Girsevich S, Ortega-Salgado A, Prieto-Patron A, Córdoba-Córdoba R, Yamazaki-Nakashimada M. Thrombotic microangiopathy involving the gallbladder as an unusual manifestation of systemic lupus erythematosus and antiphospholipid syndrome: Case report and review of the literature. *World J. Gastroenterol.*, 2006 Nov, 12(44), 7206-9.

[10] Hegarty J, Chiu DY, Middleton RJ, Haeney MM, Newstead CG, Bruce IN, Kalra PA. O'Donoghue DJ. Nephro Dial Transplant, 2006, 21, 792-5.

[11] Lee JH, No YE, Lee YJ, Hwang JY, Lee JW, Park JH. Acalculous diffuse gallbladder wall thickening in children. Pediatr. *Gastroenterol. Hepatol. Nutr.*, 2014, 17(2), 98-103.

[12] Manuel V, Pedro GM, Cordeiro LB, Miranda SM. Acute acalculous cholecystitis in systemic lupus erythematosus: a rare initial manifestation. *Rev. Bras. Reumatol.*, 2014 Mar-Apr, 56(2), 181-4.

[13] Medina F, Alaya A, Jara LJ, Becerra M, Miranda JM, Fraga A. Acute abdominal pain in systemic lupus erythematosus: the importance of early laparatomy. *Am. J. Med.,* 1997, 103, 100-5.

[14] Mendonça JA, Marques-Neto JF, Prando P, Appenzeller S. Acute acalculous cholecystitis in juvenile systemic lupus erythematosus. *Lupus*, 2009, 18(6), 561-3.

[15] Richer O, Ulinski T, Lemelle I, Ranchin B, Loirat C, Piette JC, Quartier P, Salamon R, Bader-Meunier B; French Pediatric-Onset SLE Study Group. *Ann. Rheum. Dis.*, 2007 Feb, 66(2), 174-8.

[16] Rozin A, Lorber M, Ben-Ami H, Reisner S, Kaftori, Edoute Y. Acute acalculous cholecystitis and cardiac tamponade in a patient with drug-induced lupus. *Rheumatology* (Oxford), 2001, 40, 709-11.

[17] Shin SJ, Na KS, Jung SS, Bae SC, Yoo DH, Kim SY, Kim TH. Acute acalculous cholecystitis associated with systemic lupus erythematosus with Sjogren's syndrome. *Korean J. Intern. Med.*, 2002, 17(1), 61-4.

[18] Sultan SM, Ioannou Y, Isenberg DA. A review of gastrointestinal manifestations of systemic lupus erythematosus. *Rheumatology* (Oxford), 1999, 38, 917-32.

[19] Swanepoel CR, Floyd A, Allison H, Learmonth GM, Cassidy MJ, Pascoe MD. Acute acalculous cholecystitis complicating systemic lupus erythematosus: case report and review. *Br. Med. J.* (Clin Res Ed), 1983 Jan, 286(6361), 251-2.

[20] Tu LY, Yeh KW, Chen LC, Yao TC, Ou LS, Lee WI, Huang JL. Differences in disease features between childhood-onset and adult-onset systemic lupus erythematosus patients presenting with acute abdominal pain. *Semin. arthritis Rheum.*, 2011 Apr, 40(5), 447-54.

[21] Yuan S, Lian F, Chen D, Li H, Qiu Q, Zhan Z, Ye Y, Xu H, Liang L, Yang X. Clinical features and associated factors of abdominal pain in systemic lupus erythematosus. *J. Rheumatol.*, 2013 Dec, 40(12), 2015-22.

INDEX

B

C

D

E

J

K

L

M

N

O

P

T